PREACHING PREVENTION

PERSPECTIVES ON GLOBAL HEALTH

Series editor: James L. A. Webb, Jr.

The History of Blood Transfusion in Sub-Saharan Africa,
   by William H. Schneider

Global Health in Africa: Historical Perspectives on Disease Control,
   edited by Tamara Giles-Vernick and James L. A. Webb, Jr.

*Preaching Prevention: Born-Again Christianity and the Moral Politics
of AIDS in Uganda,* by Lydia Boyd

*The Experiment Must Continue: Medical Research and Ethics in
East Africa, 1940–2014,* by Melissa Graboyes

PREACHING PREVENTION

Born-Again Christianity and the Moral
Politics of AIDS in Uganda

Lydia Boyd

Ohio University Press
Athens

Ohio University Press, Athens, Ohio 45701
ohioswallow.com
© 2015 by Ohio University Press
All rights reserved

Printed in the United States of America
Ohio University Press books are printed on acid-free paper ☉™

All photographs are by the author.

25 24 23 22 21 20 19 18 17 16 15   5 4 3 2 1

Library of Congress Cataloging-in-Publication Data

Boyd, Lydia, author.
 Preaching prevention : born-again Christianity and the moral politics of
AIDS in Uganda / Lydia Boyd.
    p. ; cm. — (Perspectives on global health)
 Includes bibliographical references and index.
 ISBN 978-0-8214-2169-7 (hc : alk. paper) — ISBN 978-0-8214-2170-3 (pb : alk. paper) —
ISBN 978-0-8214-4532-7 (pdf)
 I. Title.   II. Series: Perspectives on global health.
 [DNLM: 1. United States. President's Emergency Plan for AIDS Relief.   2. Acquired
Immunodeficiency Syndrome—prevention & control—Uganda.   3. Acquired
Immunodeficiency Syndrome—prevention & control—United States.   4. HIV
Infections—prevention & control—Uganda.   5. HIV Infections—prevention & control—
United States.   6. Christianity—Uganda.   7. Christianity—United States.   8. Health
Policy—Uganda.   9. Health Policy—United States.   10. Sexual Abstinence—Uganda.
11. Sexual Abstinence—United States. WC 503.6]
 RA643.86.U33
 362.19697'920096761—dc23
                                                            2015026459

For Dave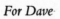

CONTENTS

ILLUSTRATIONS

Figures

Map

ACKNOWLEDGMENTS

This project has occupied me for the better part of the last decade. Over the years I have benefited from the generous support of a number of people without whom the completion of this book would have been far more difficult. My deepest debt is to the communities I studied in Uganda, especially the young adults who befriended me and spoke so frankly with me about their hopes and fears. I thank the pastor I refer to as Thomas Walusimbi, whose unique combination of charisma and candor made every day in his church an adventure. Friends and colleagues in Uganda made long periods of fieldwork away from home far more pleasurable. Two research assistants in Uganda, Consulate Guma and Susan Labwot, helped me manage the logistics of research, especially during the shorter trips I took to Uganda in 2010 and 2011; their assistance was invaluable. Besides being an especially encouraging fellow Uganda studies scholar, Holly Hanson helped me to find a wonderful house to rent during one of my longest stretches of research in Kampala. Pastor Tom Mutete gave me support at crucial junctures of this project, and offered a willing ear for discussions about Christianity in Uganda whenever I needed it. Patrick Mulindwa and the staff at the Makerere Institute of Social Research provided me with institutional support while in Uganda. I am especially grateful to the family of Edward and Esther Kimuli, who hosted me as a visiting college student in Uganda in 1998, and who have treated me as part of their extended family since then. Their daughter Catherine and their son Andrew and Andrew's wife Clare shared their homes with me during different periods of fieldwork, and their friendship has made my understanding of all aspects of Ugandan life fuller.

The primary period of fieldwork for this project was supported by a Fulbright Institute of International Education grant; I thank Dorothy Ngalombi and the late Paul Stevenson, both at the U.S. embassy in Kampala, for their help administering that grant. Other periods of fieldwork were supported by a Summer Fieldwork grant and a MacCracken Fellowship, both from New York University (NYU); and a Junior Faculty Development Grant from the University of North Carolina (UNC). A University Research Council Small Grant from UNC provided funding for the map included in chapter 2 and for the completion of the book's index. A fellowship at the Institute for the History of the Production of Knowledge (NYU) provided me with a year of support during the completion of an early draft of this book. I thank Troy Duster, Emily Martin, and Mary Poovey for that opportunity.

I am deeply indebted to the professors who guided this project in its earliest stages, most especially Tom Beidelman, Fred Myers, Bambi Schieffelin, Rayna Rapp, and Aisha Khan; their contributions to this book and to my growth as a scholar are too numerous to count. Friends and colleagues at New York University and beyond provided me with invaluable support, insight, and camaraderie: Elise Andaya, Ilka Datig, Nica Davidov, Kristin Dowell, Omri Elisha, Sholly Gunter, Jelena Karanovic, Jack Murphy, Karin Rachbauer, Pilar Rau, Ruti Talmor, and Will Thompson.

I am fortunate to have completed this book at the University of North Carolina–Chapel Hill in the company of a dynamic community of scholars. I have especially benefited from the support of my colleagues in the Department of African, African American, and Diaspora Studies—particularly my department chair Eunice Sahle. The Moral Economies of Medicine working group, hosted by members of the departments of Anthropology and Social Medicine, has been a rich forum of intellectual exchange and engagement. Special thanks to members of that group, and in particular Peter Redfield and Michele Rivkin-Fish. Two undergraduate research assistants at UNC, Mia Celnarova and Courtney Reed, helped with the transcription and coding of interviews. Friends at UNC have provided me with a supportive community in which to grapple with new ideas; very special thanks go to Mara Buchbinder, Emily Burrill, Jocelyn Chua, Jean Dennison, Jesse Summers, and Ariana Vigil. I could not imagine the process of writing this book, from beginning to end, without the support and close friendship of Ayako Takamori.

For reading and providing valuable feedback on parts of the manuscript, often at critical junctures in the writing process, I thank Emily Burrill, Nica Davidov, Michele Rivkin-Fish, Ayako Takamori, Clare Talwalker, and especially Dave Pier. For her supportive words and keen eye in the final stages of writing, I thank Holly Hanson. Two anonymous reviewers at Ohio University Press provided me with careful readings of the entire text and gave me very thoughtful insights on how to expand and improve my arguments. I am grateful to Gillian Berchowitz at Ohio University Press and Jim Webb, the editor of the Perspectives on Global Health series, for seeing potential in my manuscript.

A version of chapter 6 has been published previously in *Anthropological Quarterly* 86, no. 3 (2013) as "The Problem with Freedom: Homosexuality and Human Rights in Uganda" and is included here courtesy of the Institute for Ethnographic Research. Special thanks to Phil Schwartzberg at Meridian Mapping for the map that appears in chapter 2.

Writing a book can be an isolating process, and it is those closest to you who provide the emotional support that sees you through to the project's completion. My parents, Jean Boyd and the late Joe Boyd, were unfailing in their encouragement of me, as have been my sisters Meredith and Sarah. I am most grateful for the extraordinary love of my husband, Dave Pier, and my daughter Ivy. Ivy was born just before I finished this book, and she has brought Dave and me the unadulterated joy that comes from seeing the world through a child's curious eyes. Dave and I fell in love in Uganda, doing fieldwork alongside each other. The work that follows was made much richer because of our many discussions about Ugandan society and the experiences we shared there together. I dedicate this book to him.

INTRODUCTION

The Politics and Antipolitics of Miracles

The story of the early years of the AIDS pandemic in Uganda is now well known, but the lived experience beneath the streams of data is still hard to grasp. By the early 1990s, in some of the hardest-hit trading centers of southwestern Uganda every third household had an adult member dying of AIDS.[1] HIV prevalence rates were some of the highest in the world, nearing 15 percent of the national population.[2] Communities were faced with rates of death and disability that can only be described as devastating. Uganda, a country in eastern Africa, would soon become all but synonymous with the virus. And yet, against seemingly unimaginable odds and during a decade of intense economic and political upheaval, Ugandans were somehow able to roll back the tide of HIV/AIDS. Years before the World Health Organization was able to mobilize a global response to the epidemic, and during a decade when U.S. federal policies addressing AIDS were all but absent, Ugandans living in out-of-the-way places,[3] far from the reaches of academic biomedicine, were winning the fight against this deadly disease. Beginning in the late 1980s the seemingly inexorable spread of the virus began to slow. By the early 1990s HIV prevalence in Uganda began to drop precipitously. This reversal was so dramatic, and so unexpected, that it has been dubbed a "miracle" of HIV prevention success. By the early years of the twenty-first century, Uganda's national prevalence rate was well below 10 percent of the population, and the epicenter of the global AIDS crisis had shifted to other parts of the continent.

Uganda's "miracle" catapulted the country to the forefront of debates over HIV/AIDS prevention—debates whose stakes grew higher as global funds for treatment and prevention grew dramatically in the decades that followed. This book is about the wakes produced as this miraculous story was reclaimed, retold, used to justify certain responses to the epidemic, and adopted by politicians on both sides of the Atlantic to buttress new forms of political capital and international influence. It is a study of an American AIDS policy's reception in Uganda, and the ways in which a policy supposedly drawn from Uganda's early success returned there to shift the landscape of HIV activism and advocacy, engaging and reshaping long-standing arguments about sexual morality, marriage, and gender relations.

In 2003, President George W. Bush reversed a long period of intermittent action and partial measures by announcing a global AIDS policy of unprecedented proportions. Using soaring, optimistic language, Bush proclaimed that the President's Emergency Plan for AIDS Relief (PEPFAR) represented a "great mission of rescue" that would prevent new HIV infections and save the lives of millions living with AIDS around the world. To promote HIV treatment and prevention was to enable "the advance of freedom" itself, reasserting America as a beacon of "hope" in parts of the world wrought by the epidemic's crisis.[4] The scope of PEPFAR was indeed transformative, for the first time bringing effective treatment to millions of people living with AIDS in resource-poor countries. But PEPFAR was also controversial. Of the $3 billion reserved for HIV prevention programs in targeted countries, one-third of monies were earmarked for abstinence and faithfulness-only programs. Under PEPFAR's guidelines, these programs advocated personal "behavior change" as a frontline defense against the virus. President Bush and his advisers argued that empowering individuals to practice better self-control—by delaying sexual debut and remaining "faithful" to spouses—was the best remedy for an epidemic that had confounded public health officials worldwide. But critics in the United States and abroad viewed these stipulations as needless restrictions on aid, siphoning money away from other types of prevention programs, such as access to HIV testing, the promotion of condom use, and broad-based sexual education.[5] More pointedly, others argued that such stipulations were made solely to forward Bush's political agenda, and especially to appease his evangelical Christian supporters, who had newly embraced the AIDS epidemic as the frontline in a battle to reassert religious values in American policy making.[6]

With its emphasis on self-empowerment and personal accountability as pathways to disease management, PEPFAR dovetailed with other trends in conservative American policy making of the 1990s and the early years of the twenty-first century, a period defined by neoliberal strategies emphasizing the weakening of state welfare and the expansion of global free-market capitalism. An ethic of "self-help" pervaded policy reforms of this period, cultivating individual will and personal empathy as stand-ins for diminishing state resources.[7] Under PEPFAR the Bush administration emphasized approaches to AIDS prevention that were predicated on an individual's ability to manage and control his or her own exposure to disease risk. The term *behavior change*, which became a touchstone in debates over AIDS prevention policy during this period, was appealing to its supporters for the ways it focused attention on individual autonomy in sexual behavior. Like U.S. welfare recipients, participants in PEPFAR-funded prevention programs were compelled to become more responsible for their own care. If one could make better decisions about when and with whom one had sex—if one could abstain, or remain "faithful" in marriage—HIV risk could in theory be reduced or eliminated.

PEPFAR's "great mission of rescue" was intended to alleviate the far-off suffering of, most prominently, African victims.[8] But if PEPFAR was in part a project intent on ending the suffering wrought by the epidemic, it was also something more than a humanitarian endeavor. It was a global health program of unequaled scope, a project that sought to intervene in behaviors and beliefs about sexual relationships, medicine, and family life in order to better address the crisis. American "compassionate" sentiment helped form particular approaches to international governance and aid, approaches that were invested not only in recognizing and alleviating suffering but also in managing and "empowering" suffering populations and individuals. This American response helped outline a particular object of its care—what I call the *accountable subject*: a model for healthy behavior that, as I will discuss throughout this book, conflicted with other approaches to health and well-being in Uganda. Accountability was an approach to public health that emphasized individual responsibility for disease prevention; one that envisioned the locus of disease risk in personal behavior and choice, rather than broader structural, economic, and social factors that might also contribute to well-being. It was animated by a Western cultural orientation to health that places value on the virtues of physical autonomy and independence. In Uganda, where health has long been considered in part a function of the social and spiritual relationships one has with others, a message of self-reliance as the best pathway to healthiness had its limits.

This book considers the effects of these shifts in U.S. policy making from the point of view of the Ugandan born-again Christian AIDS activists who embraced Bush's restrictions on HIV prevention funding and celebrated what they termed a more "moral" approach to solving the problems of the epidemic. By 2004, when I began this research, Ugandan religious institutions, especially nondenominational and Pentecostal born-again churches, emerged in a way they never had before as key players in debates over AIDS prevention, seeking out newly available funds through PEPFAR to organize teach-ins advocating youth abstinence and protests against "sexual immorality." Kampala's university campuses were awash with prayer groups meditating on the value of "sexual purity." Saturday night discos competed with gospel-infused revivals where students were admonished to "keep their underwear on!" Ugandan born-again Christian arguments about what constituted moral behavior were shaped not only by President Bush's "compassionate conservative" intentions but also by long-standing debates over the nature of family and kinship obligation and the role of women in Ugandan society. Emboldened by the interest and attention of conservative American Christians, born-again churches in the capital city of Kampala became key sites where "accountability" was actualized and put to use by Ugandan youth, at times with unexpected results.

In its focus on Ugandan activists, this book takes up the adoption and implementation of a global health program by Ugandans themselves, tracking the ways international agendas are repurposed to address culturally and historically specific experiences related to gender, family, and sexuality. Public health programs, especially those like PEPFAR, which are concerned with the intimacy of family life and sexuality, are programs that forward powerful moral claims about what it means to act healthily. The seemingly unassailable ethics that underlie dominant approaches to global health today—particularly ideals like accountability—are never neutral. There is, to echo the anthropologist James Ferguson, a "politics and anti-politics" to global health miracles.[9] That is, humanitarian projects like PEPFAR claim a moral imperative that seems to place it outside the realm of politics. To alleviate suffering is ostensibly an act beyond political motive, even as the compassionate sentiments that underlie such projects help shape particular approaches to governance. The story of Uganda's early AIDS prevention success was a product of this antipolitical humanitarian realm: embraced as a politically disinterested story of human triumph even as it was used to buttress and validate certain approaches to care and humanitarian relief, approaches that worked to create particular kinds of subjects for American compassion.

If this is a story about the ways a health policy travels, it is also a study of how African recipients of a public health program took up and transformed a lesson about accountability, emphasizing both the appeal and the limitations of a global approach to AIDS prevention. PEPFAR was a policy that circulated, from its roots in Uganda's early success to its formation in the United States, and back again; and with each iteration it was adopted and used by both Americans and Ugandans to forward their own ideas about the benefits of accountability, self-control, and "moral" behavior. PEPFAR's emphasis on "behavior change" reflects the dominant ethos underlying approaches to humanitarian care and global health today, but it was, on the ground, an approach that was contested in practice, reshaped by Ugandan orientations to moral behavior and well-being that conflicted with the American ideal of "accountability." In this sense, the story of PEPFAR challenges the unidirectional image of global health: one in which Western countries create and fund programs outlining models for care and healthiness and Africans simply adopt such models.

In the following chapters I explore how "behavior change"—with its particular emphasis on an ideal of personal accountability—was an approach to prevention that was formed by a historical moment in the United States and Africa. It was an approach characterized by neoliberal economic policies that emphasized the individual—rather than the state, kin group, or community— as the central agent in processes of development and social transformation. The shape of the "accountable subject" is evident everywhere now, from messages like PEPFAR's, in which the self-controlled, abstaining individual is the key to disease management, to rural development projects where, as Tania Li has argued, individual will drives social improvement schemes.[10] In Uganda, neoliberal policies have reorganized institutional and state apparatuses, but they have also effected changes in the experience of moral personhood and the evaluation of moral conduct. What sorts of subjects are made legible by approaches to governance that demand that subjects become more "accountable" for their care, and with what consequences?

The larger impact of humanitarian aid and global politics was felt not only in the presence of PEPFAR's programs but in the changing nature of Ugandan society, where older values predicated on the interdependence of youth and elders were being challenged by discourses emphasizing an "entrepreneurial" spirit and the benefits of young people's initiative and independence. "Accountability" was a discourse that stoked deep tensions over the costs and benefits of such changes to society. Young adults felt these tensions keenly as they struggled to imagine their own futures and families. Uganda's born-again churches were at the center of these transformations, adopting a message of personal "success" and moral asceticism in the face of a rapidly changing social environment—where everything from gender equality to conspicuous displays of wealth provoked moral rebuke and concerns about the state of Ugandan culture and values.

These broader shifts in AIDS prevention and activism have affected experiences of health and well-being in Uganda. The emergent emphasis on individual will and personal agency helped reinforce a new and distinct way of being an ethical sexual subject in Uganda—one that diverged from other messages about moral conduct that existed alongside it. In Uganda, as in many African societies, the liberal ideal of the rational, autonomous person that animates so many modern institutions and values—from Western biomedicine to the project of human rights to the ideal of accountability itself—coexists with other models for personhood, and especially those that construe the person as defined not by the qualities of interiority and autonomy but instead by experiences of social interdependence and obligation to others. In Uganda, relationships of interdependence between members of kin groups and between patrons and clients are critical ways social actors constitute their place in the world, and forge a moral and social identity. Ugandan experiences of personhood were in many ways counterposed to the message of individual accountability and independence that the PEPFAR program promoted.

In Uganda, these older models for moral personhood became critical touchpoints in debates over the concept of accountability as both a mode of prevention and a model for behavior. PEPFAR's emphasis on accountability could provoke dilemmas for Ugandan young adults, who were also taught that their assertion of independence, especially through their withdrawal from social and sexual relationships, could in certain instances be viewed as dangerous, immoral, or antisocial. In southern Uganda, where the pursuit of health has been characterized by one historian as a "collective endeavor,"[11] how did people make sense of a message that emphasized autonomy in decisions about sex and wellness? This book concerns itself with these sorts of conflicts: What does it mean to speak of a "self-empowering" approach to health care? What sort of moral agency is being advanced by an emphasis on choice and self-control? How did young Ugandans navigate the underlying conflicts inherent in the message of accountability? And, most significantly, how did this message come to affect the politics and experiences of health, disease, and family life in Ugandan communities?

The argument of this book is twofold. The first part is that *the accountable subject* reflects a particular approach to governance that has come to dominate contemporary frameworks for global health. Today in Uganda, as in much of the world where humanitarianism is at work, demonstrating a will to improve is the way one becomes a visible subject for nongovernmental endeavors. In this new model, one's claim to certain services—access to clean water, education, health care—is no longer the rights-based claim of a citizen, nor a claim rooted in forms of traditional community-based obligation. Rather, access to humanitarian and nonstate aid becomes dependent on one's ability to demonstrate accountability for one's condition, to be a good subject of compassion, and to be able to harness the will *to be improved* by a donor's humanitarian attentions.[12]

The second and more prolonged argument of this book is that this approach to health and healing is animated by particular moral sentiments and ethical dispositions that are contested in practice. Decisions about health are broached as moral conflicts, and to understand the effects of a global policy like PEPFAR we need to better understand the diverse models for moral agency and personhood that define the pursuit of health in particular settings. In Uganda, the values that inhabited accountability—to be autonomous, self-sufficient—were experienced in tension with other ways of being that were also understood to define the experience of health. Health in Uganda was not expressed solely as the good management of one's interior, physical state. Moral and physical well-being depended also on the proper management of one's obligations to and relationships with others—relationships that were believed to directly affect one's physical and mental state. If Americans attempted to forward an authoritative model of proper, healthy behavior marked by the emphasis placed on the virtue of being accountable for one's own well-being, Ugandans engaged this message on more uncertain terrain. The rest of this introduction elaborates on these points and provides background information on the community where my research was conducted. I begin with a discussion of how and why accountability has come to dominate global approaches to health today.

The Accountable Subject:
Biopolitical Aid and the Effects of Compassion

When I write about the "accountable subject" I mean to draw attention to a particular way of thinking about good and proper conduct—conduct that is thought to produce healthiness and prosperity and has come into focus in recent years in part through policies like PEPFAR. PEPFAR's faith in individuals' capacity to change—to reform their behaviors—formed the core of its policy directives.[13] It was rooted in an underlying belief that both moral good and socioeconomic good follow from the actualization of ideals like independence, autonomy, and personal freedom. And it differs from other popular approaches to disease management—for instance, methods that encourage technological interventions, such as an increase in serostatus testing or the development of a vaccine, or methods that encourage structural changes that address socioeconomic or other inequalities linked to health risk, such as gender differentials in education or high rates of domestic violence. PEPFAR emphasized only one type of prevention approach in its funding stipulations, requiring that one-third of monies directed to prevention, US$1 billion, be used for "abstinence and faithfulness" education. So why—and why *now*—have the ideals of self-control and personal accountability come to govern public health regimes, especially those concerned with AIDS prevention?

An ethic of self-regulation seems to have intensified in recent years alongside changes to dominant forms of state and international governance. Beginning in the 1980s, two interrelated trends began to shift the field of economic development—and in turn, health care—in Uganda: the first was the expanding influence of a neoliberal economic doctrine, and the second was the emergence of a humanitarian ethos as a core component of transnational aid. To understand the present meaning of "accountability," it is necessary to understand the ways in which it is a message shaped by these intersecting trends in global governance.

Neoliberalism is a term that has itself been the object of criticism for the ways it is often characterized as a monolithic global force by social scientists, a term whose meaning, in its all-encompassing influence, has become ambiguous.[14] Neoliberalism might be most succinctly defined as a set of economic policies that came to dominate the spheres of transnational aid and global restructuring in the 1980s. The structural adjustment programs advocated by the World Bank and the International Monetary Fund, and adopted by aid-recipient countries like Uganda, included provisions that sought to "rebalance" a country's economy, usually by recommending various fiscal austerity measures, including the deregulation of industry, privatization, and the lowering of tax burdens for foreign investment.

Scholarly interest in neoliberalism has concerned itself with the social and political effects of these economic measures, and especially the ways this particular brand of economic calculation has transformed approaches to governance.[15] Building on the earlier work of Michel Foucault,[16] these authors have focused attention on the ways a certain type of economic rationality has come to encompass aspects of life previously considered outside the domain of the market. David Harvey's oft-cited assessment defines neoliberalism by the core assumption that "individual freedoms are guaranteed by freedom of the market and of trade."[17] Nikolas Rose similarly argues that neoliberalism cultivates an approach to governance that reconceptualizes social behavior "along economic lines—as calculative actions undertaken through the universal human faculty of choice."[18] In this schema, rational choice is imbued with a moral value. Proper conduct is outlined by the ability to self-regulate and make "productive" choices. If people are "freed" to choose for themselves, they will learn to better govern and self-regulate their conduct.

Given this emphasis on rational choice, projects of development and economic restructuring in the neoliberal state have come to emphasize the individual, rather than the state or community, as the central actor in projects of social transformation.[19] Daromir Rudnyckyj, writing about similar economic changes in Indonesia, calls this period the "afterlife of development," an era marked by the shift from state-sanctioned investment to an era in which "this duty is transferred to the citizens themselves," who are made to feel both more empowered and also more accountable for state services that may no longer be taken for granted.[20] It is this aspect of neoliberalism that interests me. What happens when the pursuit of health in a place like Uganda is viewed through the lens of the rational individual decision maker?

The realms of biomedicine and public health may be particularly fruitful arenas in which to explore this emergent emphasis on individual accountability. Foucault's lectures on "biopolitics" have highlighted the ways the physical body have become a more explicit focus of governance in the modern era.[21] Biopower, according to Foucault, is enacted both in the policies that manage populations (such as those that regulate reproduction and population growth) and in the new ways individuals are taught to regulate and manage the body itself. More recently, scholars have proposed concepts such as "biological" and "therapeutic" citizenship to describe how biology and physical need have become key resources through which individuals stake claims to state and nonstate resources.[22] If the body has become a more explicit focus for rights and regulations, it is also now increasingly conceived of as an optimizable resource.[23] We are taught not only that we are responsible for ourselves but that our bodies and our experiences of physical health are the means through which we may improve and become more responsible citizens. As perhaps they have never been before, our bodies are the means by which we are governed and learn to govern ourselves.

When I note that PEPFAR's key prevention message of "abstinence and faithfulness" may be analyzed as biopolitical sexual discourse and practice, I

The Politics and Antipolitics of Miracles

mean to draw attention to the sorts of ethical dispositions that abstinence and sexual self-regulation were supposed to generate: the intense focus on individual conduct as a site of economic and social transformation. In Uganda, particularly in the churches where my research was based, abstinence and marital faithfulness were spoken of as embodied practices believed to make people not only more moral but more economically successful; more "intentional" in decisions about work, family, and relationships; and more accountable for their mistakes. Abstinence and marital faithfulness were believed to cultivate a new, more productive young adult, empowered to embrace her own potential, more self-reliant, autonomous, and "invested" in herself. This rationalization of conduct was undertaken often at the expense of other ways of addressing social crisis: through forms of community organizing or large-scale structural changes to government or state. The "accountable subject" reflects these particular ideas about health and wellness, the ways that Ugandans in the early years of the new century were being taught, and at times were refiguring, a message that told them they could be empowered by making better personal choices about their bodies and avoiding the risks associated with disease and infection.

If neoliberal rationality and new forms of biological governance have given shape to the present-day onus on personal accountability, the accountable subject has also emerged in tandem with a particular humanitarian ethos that has refigured international aid and the relationship between Africa and the West. The changes that followed the adoption of structural adjustment in Uganda may be most noticeable in the mechanisms that organize aid and relief operations in Uganda. In President Yoweri Museveni's first decade in power, international donor aid to Uganda expanded more than tenfold.[24] But beginning in the 1980s, donor countries increasingly sought to shift grants away from state-led development programs and toward a development sector dominated by nongovernmental organizations. The privatization of aid has been swift and dramatic in places like Uganda. Between 1990 and 1998 the total amount of aid managed by nongovernmental organizations (NGOs) in Africa more than tripled, from US$1 billion to US$3.5 billion.[25] During a similar period the World Bank saw a fourfold increase in the percentage of its projects managed by NGOs, from less than 10 percent in 1990 to more than 40 percent in 2001.[26]

International aid has not only been directed toward a more diffuse, privatized sector but has also increasingly been defined to address "humanitarian," rather than explicitly political or economic, needs. The pursuit of health in the Global South has been especially affected by such shifts. HIV/AIDS, an epidemic of unprecedented proportions, has caused a state of crisis that demands immediate intervention. Health is imagined in this context not as a project of optimization, as it is in wealthy countries, but as one of exception. Humanitarianism may be distinguished from other historical and philosophical approaches to transnational aid by its explicit concern with human suffering. In the humanitarian state, physical need is the central recourse through which citizens and others make claims to scarce therapeutic resources and other forms of government care.[27] This state of crisis creates a differential in treatment that distinguishes experiences of health and disease in places like Uganda from those in the Global North. Anthropologists Miriam Ticktin and Vinh-Kim Nguyen have argued that the act of linking aid to a demonstration of acute physical distress is problematic because the very exceptionality of this state closes off other ways of advocating for rights and access to care. In his study of AIDS treatment programs in West Africa, Nguyen asks, "What forms of politics might emerge in a world where the only way to survive is to have a fatal illness?"[28] What does it mean to view health as a state of exception, and health care as a practice pursued through a lens of "experimentality," a term Adriana Petryna uses to point to the inequalities that shape global health and medical research?[29] The global health industry—which extends beyond humanitarian aid to include medical research, a realm where seemingly marginal and unregulated, yet needy, populations like those in sub-Saharan Africa figure prominently as test cases[30]—has helped refashion what it means to be healthy, and how healthiness is sought out, in places like Uganda. The accountable subject is also a product of these developments, where healthiness is pursued on paths of limited resources, and where the ability to demonstrate need, and become an "appropriate" subject of care, matters most.

Both neoliberal governance and humanitarian compassion helped shape new ways of thinking about being a good, proper, and moral person in Kampala. But as may already be apparent, the terms *compassion* and *accountability* are embedded in particular frameworks for understanding persons and agency that were far from universal in Uganda. A key tension that surrounded the adoption of behavior change emerged from its difference from—and occasional overlap with—other ways of acting as a good, productive, and moral person. As I will discuss throughout this book, the practices attributed to being an accountable subject were contested, emerging as an assemblage of global policy and local moral subjectivities that reshaped

Ugandan orientations to health and well-being in the years following PEPFAR's adoption.

Morality and Public Health

The first part of this book's argument, which I have outlined above, is that PEPFAR is a policy defined by the conjuncture of neoliberal economic forms and an emergent humanitarian ethos in international aid, which together have helped outline the accountable subject at the center of global health. The second part of this argument is that the neoliberal concern with accountability is one animated by moral sentiments that were contested in practice. Public health programs, especially those that seek to prevent disease, are projects that intercede in broader moral debates, creating models for behavior that outline individuals' responsibilities to themselves and to each other. The message that PEPFAR forwarded—to become more accountable for one's health by avoiding HIV/AIDS—was a choice that was constrained by a number of economic and social factors. But abstaining, and becoming accountable, was also a choice that was viewed as a pathway to being a certain type of (moral) person in Uganda. Throughout this book I consider how decisions about health are often experienced as moral conflicts that highlight competing models for how to be good, healthy, and successful. To better understand the ways public health messages are interpreted in varied cultural settings, we need to be better able to recognize the role of diverse models for moral agency and personhood in the pursuit of health and wellness.

When I use the term *public health*, I refer specifically to the Western discipline familiar to most readers, under which a program for AIDS prevention, like those supported by PEPFAR, might fall. But the term also relates to a broader category of projects encompassed by the terms *social health* and *public healing*,[31] which have been used to describe African practices of healing as collective endeavors, ones that are at the center of projects to maintain and secure social welfare. Neil Kodesh's study of public healing rituals in precolonial Buganda has highlighted the ways that such rituals emphasized the connections between "a community's moral economy and continued well-being."[32] Studies of healing in Africa have long underscored how practices that seek to manage health extend beyond addressing the physical ailments of suffering individuals to consider the broader social and moral context of health and prosperity.[33] In communities across Africa, people's relationships with each other, with a spiritual realm, and with their environments have long been factors that were considered to shape and intervene in experiences of health and illness. Even as there is much to distinguish modern public health projects from this longer history of African public healing, both sorts of projects attempt to forward a notion of social order that is predicated on specific moral orientations and sets of obligations.[34] Modern public health projects set out to teach people to subordinate their personal desires and interests for the broader public good: "Cover your mouth when you sneeze." "Kitchen workers must wash their hands before returning to work." Public health programs are also projects that seek to inculcate models for healthy behavior within the public or social (and moral) context that gives our experiences of healthiness and social obligation shape.

Given this broader context, this book explores what a more explicit consideration of morality might bring to our understanding of health, and of global health programs in particular. To understand how AIDS prevention messages were engaged by Ugandan youth, we need to understand not just how health and well-being are linked to clinical practices or evaluations of physical risk but also the ways health is also a product of "moral imaginings and moral expressions."[35] Our moral perspective on the world, or what the anthropologist T. O. Beidelman has called our "moral imagination," is the frame through which our experiences of sickness and healing—in fact, the entirety of our social world—is defined and coped with.[36] A central aspect of the human experience is the way we confront uncertainty through practices of moral reflection: we imagine and speculate about others' and our own pain and suffering. Our moral imagination also provides us with the ability to "scrutinize, contemplate and judge" our world,[37] to imagine what is and what might be different. It may be understood to "map the ambiguity of social experience";[38] it is how we make sense of uncertainty and change. Perhaps because of this, anthropologists' interest in the topic of morality has focused in particular on the problems of navigating and making sense of radical social changes. In several recent ethnographies, the study of morality has provided a way of understanding and analyzing the contradictions between indigenous ways of life and the ethical orientations associated with modernity.[39] This has been especially true of studies of contemporary Islam and Christianity.[40] Christian conversion has been noted for the ways in which it can precipitate a radical reconfiguration of social and cultural forms, marked especially by a sense of discontinuity between older values predicated on social cohesion and interdependence, and a modern-Christian emphasis on the value of individual agency, moral interiority, and personal autonomy.[41]

As much as social changes and social crises (such as the AIDS epidemic) have elicited a sense of disjuncture and discontinuity, in practice such conflicts are almost never experienced as linear and distinct.[42] One benefit of a focus on the ways people engage moral norms is that it provides us with a more nuanced understanding of how individuals make sense of social changes and the competing values attributed to different ways of being.[43] The crisis surrounding AIDS and its prevention is addressed on such moral terms in Uganda not so much as a problem of right and wrong, or as a problem addressed through the dictates of a certain religious doctrine or biomedical decree, but on terms that seek to define and establish the outlines of personhood and moral obligation. In the communities where I worked, I found that the American emphasis on accountable behavior was taken up and transformed by youth as they pursued multiple, often contradictory, messages about how to be good, healthy persons. As much as abstinence seemed to emphasize a neoliberal focus on the individual, in practice it also reinforced other, older models for sexual subjecthood. For instance, as I discuss in chapter 4, Ugandan youth viewed abstinence as something more than the cultivation of self-control and personal responsibility. They also viewed abstinence through frameworks for spiritual and community well-being that emphasized the strength of an individual's relationships with others. As an embodied practice, abstinence (along with its partner message, faithfulness) mediated between the seemingly opposed experiences of autonomy and interdependence in neoliberal Uganda and the cultural and ethical meanings that lay beneath both ideals. A focus on the moral conflicts that are rooted in neoliberal approaches to governance and global aid provides us with a better understanding of the effects of such policies and of the role of African subjects in implementing and transforming these projects.

In the pages that follow I consider how health is pursued as a component of moral personhood and explore abstinence and marital faithfulness as ethical practices—or, following Foucault, "technologies of the self" by which young Ugandans sought to make themselves into certain kinds of moral persons. Foucault's notion of ethical practice—that ethics is a matter of self-cultivation governed by practical "techniques" that guide conduct—has proved valuable to anthropologists because it establishes an understanding of ethics that emphasizes the quotidian practices that generate culturally variable ethical and moral subjects.[44] Such analysis allows us to understand moral behaviors and choices not only as products of sovereign will governed by Kantian reason but also as actions shaped by variable forms of social power.

In this schema, ethical practice may be analyzed as generative of multiple experiences of personhood, not dependent on a privileging of the autonomous post-Enlightenment individual.[45]

This is a focus that allows for a more nuanced understanding of the effects of public health policies that are enacted within diverse social and cultural frameworks and by persons who are motivated by multiple models of health and moral agency. This approach also enables us to explore how moral practices may be challenged, and how two overlapping moral systems may be navigated by social actors. In Uganda, the outlines of the accountable subject were encountered by youth in and through their efforts to abstain and be faithful, but these practices were complicated by efforts to manage competing models for personhood and competing outlines of what it meant to be successful and ethical in Kampala today. Only by understanding the underlying logics and moral orientations that Ugandan youth brought to the practice of abstinence can we fully understand the limits and possibilities that the message "abstain and be faithful to avoid HIV/AIDS" might have—in Uganda and elsewhere.

Moral Authorities: Born-Again Churches and Social Protest in Uganda

In Uganda the moral conflicts that surround AIDS prevention have been shaped by broader changes to Ugandan society since the 1980s. The epidemic coincided, as it did on much of the African continent, with a period of rapid urbanization that precipitated widespread alterations to social bonds. Family relationships were especially burdened by the epidemic, as exceedingly high rates of death and disability forced people to rely on extended relationships of kin and community in order to cope. But the changing nature of these same relationships—as young adults delayed marriage and women left their natal homes to find wage labor—also stoked concerns that the abandonment of "traditional" values was a cause of the disease and society's misfortune. "Loose women" and "unruly youth" were a frequent target of blame for the virus in Uganda, as they were elsewhere.[46] Because it became associated for many—especially elders—with changing family dynamics and the perceived misbehaviors attributed to newly more independent women and young adults, the epidemic intensified questions about what types of persons are morally correct in Ugandan society and about the social costs of both modern and traditional ways of being. These practices of reflection have especially engaged the spiritual realm, and blame for sexual misconduct has in some instances,

The Politics and Antipolitics of Miracles

as Heike Behrend has recounted in her study of Western Uganda,[47] been attributed to occult forces at work in society. High rates of death during the epidemic fueled a sense of intense social, moral, and spiritual insecurity.

This sense of insecurity has also been exacerbated by the instability of the promises of new forms of global governance and political economy in neoliberal Uganda. Ugandans today live during an era when material wealth is both more visible and far out of reach for most people. The youth I studied, who lived in Uganda's largest city and who were mostly enrolled or recently graduated from the country's most prestigious university, regularly expressed a sense of frustration with their prospects for success despite their relatively privileged positions. Levels of unemployment were extremely high, and youth were forced to depend for extended periods on their parents and other elders for support. There was a growing sense of ambivalence about both an older generation's emphasis on traditional social obligations and the modern emphasis on personal empowerment and individualism inherent in policies like PEPFAR.

It was into this environment that a born-again movement to prevent AIDS took shape in Uganda. The growth of a religiously oriented AIDS activism in the early years of the twenty-first century points to the expanding importance of spirituality as a mode of social critique in neoliberal Africa. A number of scholars have emphasized the ways that criticisms of contemporary conditions by Africans are taking new forms, focused less on tangible actors and more often now articulated through the "sacrificial logic" of Pentecostal and occult imaginaries.[48] Such analysis challenges assumptions about the oppositional relationships between faith and reason, and religion and politics, to uncover how the spiritual realm has become a critical field in which Africans engage the problem of the moral uncertainty of political power. Spirituality is central to our understanding of how young adults in Uganda manage the contemporary sense of material and physical crisis, the tension and ambivalence that characterizes the neoliberal promise of self-help, and the behavioral ideal of accountability.

My interest in the world of born-again Christianity is with the ways such communities provided a model not only for moral behavior but for "moral ambitions" and ways of effecting or responding to social change that many Ugandans found objectionable.[49] Omri Elisha, in his study of socially engaged evangelical Americans, uses the term "moral ambitions" to "draw attention to the intrinsic sociality of such aspirations . . . their inexorable orientation toward other people and their inalienability from social networks and institutions."[50] In Uganda, moral ambitions have long played a central role in the politics of the colonial and postcolonial state. In his recent history of colonial protest in eastern Africa, Derek Peterson argues that mid-twentieth-century political innovation was not centered in the struggle for democratic rights and independence but instead in the moral arguments that engaged anxieties related to changes in intergenerational and gender relations.[51] Arguments over women's newfound independence and youths' perceived unruliness became ways for men to reassert their moral authority and to take control of a narrative of historical change. Like Elisha, I see the support of abstinence as an ambitious project engaged in by born-again youth, one through which they sought to enact ethical reform on themselves and, in the process, to transform society.

In this way, this book engages broader questions about the meaning and effect of a seemingly expanding religiosity in the modern world. Far from Max Weber's prediction of a "disenchantment" with belief, Ugandans and Americans alike have embraced new and old forms of religious practice to make sense of, and even forward, a neoliberal emphasis on rationality and self-help. PEPFAR was a policy that sought to transform the ways communities and governments responded to social problems by seeking to funnel money to community and religious organizations directly and by targeting faith as a basis of social transformation. By focusing on a community of religious activists who responded to PEPFAR's call to action, this study illuminates something about the role of religious practice in contemporary international aid. I examine churches as places where politics happens in mundane but transformative ways: in lessons about sex, family, and marriage; and in the support of certain types of relationships over others. In this broader sense this study builds on questions about American evangelicalism and social activism today, but places these questions in a very different social and historical context than that of the United States—one governed by quite distinct models and orientations toward religiosity, sociality, and morality.

This study also takes up questions about the nature and effect of the financial and personal relationships between American and Ugandan Christians. Since the 1970s, American Christians have become more active in political issues and social activism, a historical shift that has drawn extensive scholarly interest.[52] But their efforts to engage Africans and others in their political projects—efforts that have become increasingly important to American Christian communities—have thus far received less scholarly attention. The recent controversy over Uganda's antihomosexuality legislation, which

I address in chapter 6, drew popular attention to the depth and impact that such intercontinental religious ties may have. My interest is not in the Americans who become involved in African affairs by donating money to churches, by supporting or withdrawing support for legislative efforts like the recent Anti-Homosexuality Act in Uganda, or by traveling in groups to volunteer in Ugandan communities. My concerns are instead with how American Christian perspectives are taken up and transformed by Ugandans themselves.

Research Methods and Fieldwork Engagements

I began field research for this book in July 2004, just months after the PEPFAR program began to disseminate funds to program partners in Uganda. I first became interested in PEPFAR after I spent that month interviewing North American missionaries about their work in the development sector. The PEPFAR program, and AIDS prevention and care work, emerged as a frequent topic in discussions with these missionaries, who were newly motivated by the program to respond to the AIDS crisis. Their newfound interest in the epidemic raised questions for me about the impact of PEPFAR and the meaning of the expanding influence and involvement of Christian communities in AIDS prevention work in Africa. When I returned to conduct fieldwork in October 2005, I based my research in Ugandan church communities that were involved in promoting youth abstinence in Kampala. One church, University Hill Church (UHC), became the focus of my fieldwork and is featured prominently in this ethnography. Two other churches where I spent time are not described at length in this book, though my experiences there and the interviews I conducted with youth in those churches have contributed to the analyses I include here. One church identified as Pentecostal and the other two as nondenominational, though all belonged to the family of born-again churches that Ugandans consider distinct from the mainline mission churches—Anglican and Catholic—that have been dominant religious institutions in the country since the colonial era.

UHC was located near the Wandegeya neighborhood in Kampala and served a mostly English-speaking population. This is significant because English-language-dominant churches catered to a more educated, and thus elite, population than churches that primarily used one of Uganda's indigenous languages. This was a church that had been positioned to serve a growing population of educated urban youth in Kampala, and many members of UHC were drawn from the city's university campuses, especially nearby

Makerere University. While the church comprised a multiethnic Ugandan community, the culture of the Ganda ethnic group dominated,[53] in part because the church was led by a Ganda pastor and in part because the church itself, like the city of Kampala, is located in Buganda. For this reason, in this book I draw on literature from throughout the region to describe Ugandan cultural attitudes and orientations, but I sustain a focus, especially in the historical analysis I provide in chapter 2, on the literature of southern Uganda and especially Buganda.

UHC, as well as other churches I visited and spent time in, was actively involved in AIDS prevention activities. Over the course of my fieldwork, UHC sponsored and organized abstinence education projects, including public marches, concerts, workshops, and outreach and counseling programs. UHC was also the recipient of a modest amount of PEPFAR funding, which was received via a church-founded NGO that had been named the recipient of a grant for abstinence education. Because of the relatively sensitive nature of my research topic—which touches on spirituality, sexual relationships, and disease—both interviewee names and the names of churches remain pseudonymous for reasons of confidentiality.[54] I will describe UHC more fully in chapter 3.

For nineteen months between October 2005 and May 2007, I spent time in these communities, interviewing pastors and youth and attending services, workshops community events, prayer meetings, and women's meetings. I also lived for nine months in the home of a Ugandan family who were members of a born-again church I visited regularly, and I attended home Bible study groups and family meetings with them. (I later rented for a year a small house adjacent to the home of another member of the same church.) I returned in July 2010 and June 2011 to conduct follow-up interviews with pastors and youth. I also spent time during those visits attending parenthood workshops at UHC, where I learned more about the church's expectations for family life. I conducted group interviews with both church members and Ugandans outside the born-again community that focused on the issue of homosexuality and Uganda's 2009 Anti-Homosexuality Bill, a topic I take up in chapter 6.

I interviewed four dozen young adults and reinterviewed ten of them at least twice over the six years of primary field research, tracking how their attitudes about marriage, sexuality, and their desire for and struggles with parenthood and family life changed over time. I also interviewed eight pastors and church leaders about their hopes for their church, their involvement with AIDS prevention and activism, and their problems with church financing. I knew many more young adults, older adults, and clergy less formally, and spoke with them at church meetings and social events about their concerns in life. In addition to ethnographic fieldwork and interviews, I also interviewed individuals involved in AIDS prevention outside these churches, including people involved in advocacy and research from various other sectors including academia, the secular NGO world, and the mainline Catholic and Anglican churches.

I was positioned as a researcher within the church community I studied, though—especially by those I lived with and knew well—I was also considered a friend. The intimacy of the ethnographic encounter can be both tremendously rewarding and challenging, as frustrating as it is illuminating: it is a mode of research that generates close personal ties between researchers and research participants. Ethnographers depend on the intimacy of the fieldwork experience to help reveal deeper cultural understandings: How do people in this community think? What matters to them? As Clifford Geertz has famously described, ethnography is akin to "thick description"; it is the way we come to understand the difference between the proverbial wink and a twitch of the eye.[55]

In recent years, especially as the work of religious activists in Uganda has generated more controversy (see especially chapter 6), many people have asked me what it was like to conduct fieldwork within this community. Studying Ugandans who have embraced a version of the religiosity—born-again Christianity—that many (Ugandans and Americans alike) view as native to my own country certainly presented its own unique challenges. The church where I conducted fieldwork had relationships with Christians in the West, and so the presence of an American in church was not all that unusual. As a researcher rather than a missionary-volunteer I was, of course, positioned differently from most of these other visitors. (I am not a born-again Christian, for one thing.) Yet as many other anthropologists who have studied Christianity around the world have also noted, my position outside the "frame of belief" was not a point of particular concern or contention for the Ugandans I knew.[56] As a participant-observer I was taken seriously as someone who sought to better hear and understand the Ugandan Christian way of life. Church members took time to explain their mode of worship, their attitudes and beliefs, in part because this was the work of being a Christian—of both proselytizing and experiencing their own faith.

I was not only viewed as a potential convert (as all nonbelievers are), however; I was taken seriously as an anthropologist. This was somewhat surprising to me, as anthropology is not a discipline that is widely studied in Uganda (though, like foreign missionaries, the peripatetic academic researcher is a known commodity in Kampala). Thomas Walusimbi, the head pastor at UHC, once told a room full of church members that he wanted to start a college radio station and feature on it a show about "anthropology and our culture." Though surprising, his idea was not all that far-fetched. The study of culture—especially as it was understood in Uganda to mean "traditional culture"—was a project of some significance to a community that sought to both embrace and reform aspects of so-called traditional life. Pastor Walusimbi even once spoke to me, unprompted, about the "anthropology of the Baganda," forwarding his own analysis of the ways precolonial Ganda political relationships influence contemporary mind-sets. As a discipline concerned with understanding both the similarities and the differences between Ugandan and American Christians, anthropology presented a certain utility to the pastor. As I discuss in chapter 1, he was concerned with highlighting the agency of Africans in a world that seemed defined by the politico-economic relationships of development aid that positioned Africans as passive recipients; thus, a project focused on a deeper understanding of African actors was one he could get behind.

That being said, it was not always easy to observe and seek to understand views that were not only different from my own but at times objectionable and unsettling to me. The most challenging portions of my fieldwork were those toward the end of my study, when an antihomosexuality agenda came to dominate church activities. Both within and outside the church, discussion of homosexuality in Uganda revolved around often disturbing and violent imagery. Attacks on people accused of being gay or lesbian were becoming more common in Kampala in the wake of 2009's antihomosexuality legislation. But it was during this period that I was also struck by the way Ugandans (and especially Ugandan Christians) were being portrayed by the Western media. They have become, to use a phrase coined by the anthropologist Susan Harding, a "repugnant cultural other" in the eyes of a supposedly enlightened West.[57] Their views on homosexuality have been dismissed as either grossly misguided, a symptom of their lingering "traditionalism," or—worse yet—a reflection of their position as pawns of a sinister contingent of rogue Western conservative religious activists. Throughout my fieldwork I was struck by this persistent assumption: that Ugandan Christian social activism is pursued under the guidance of American Christians and conservative politicians and that the beliefs and interests of these two groups—American

The Politics and Antipolitics of Miracles

and Ugandan—were interchangeable. One of the main purposes of this book is to elucidate the ways this was often not the case. My intent is to reveal and explain something about the motivations and moral orientations of Ugandan Christians, highlighting their own agency and agenda in the social protests (for abstinence as an AIDS prevention method, and against homosexual rights) that have come to define them in recent years.

The Book's Structure, and an Outline of the Chapters

This book is structured as an ethnographic study of a policy in that it considers, to quote Catrin Evans and Helen Lambert, "how interventions enter into existing life worlds and both shape and are shaped by them."[58] It is divided into three sections that lead the reader from the historical and political context that gave rise to PEPFAR's origins, to an analysis of its impact within one Ugandan community, to the long-term effects or "wakes" that have remained in the years following its initial implementation. Part 1 draws on archival research, analysis of U.S. congressional records, and interviews with key figures in Uganda's health and religious sectors involved in early AIDS prevention efforts. Part 2 is the ethnographic heart of the book, where Ugandan responses to and interpretations of PEPFAR's policy are analyzed. Part 3 is also primarily ethnographic, focusing on the broader social and political effects of the policy in Uganda, especially in terms of attitudes surrounding gender and sexuality, including homosexuality.

Part 1, which outlines the context for the PEPFAR program, begins with a focus on the history of the PEPFAR policy itself and its initial implementation in Uganda. Chapter 1 explores the meaning of the idea of compassion in American politics and how it came to refigure international aid under the Bush administration. It provides a historical overview of AIDS prevention policy in Uganda and analyzes the role that born-again Christian activists have played in AIDS policy since 2004 in Kampala. It also sheds light on the motivations of the American politicians who crafted the policy and stipulated the controversial limits on how prevention programs would be funded. Chapter 2 provides historical background for the current political and religious climate in Uganda, its purpose being to focus a historical lens on the role that Christian churches have played in political and social struggles in Uganda over the course of the last century. The AIDS epidemic has heightened a sense of social instability, and in its wake there has been a proliferation of discourses that assert a return to the moral certainty promised by "traditional" gender relations, generational obligations, and modes of spiritual and social authority.

This chapter explores how these arguments have been formed in dialogue with a much longer history of debates over changing household dynamics, women's roles in society, and the place of ethnicity within the nation-state. Here I develop more fully what role so-called moral authority has played in the Ugandan political sphere and how contemporary discussions of morality are shaped by a decades-long history of the "moral reform" of the home.

Part 2 comprises chapters 3–5, which examine the meaning and practice of abstinence and faithfulness within a community of Ugandan born-again Christians. These chapters highlight how this message was refigured within Uganda to address the particular moral and spiritual struggles that young people encountered. Chapter 3 is the first of two chapters to examine the message of abstinence. The chapter focuses on how abstinence was framed as a certain type of (Christian, neoliberal) moral message and the ways it was compared and contrasted with other forms of sexual education in Uganda that emphasized different types of moral subjecthood. It includes an examination of how youth made sense of and resolved the moral disjunctures that abstinence created, and how such negotiations both established the strategy's appeal and demarcated its limitations as a public health approach. Chapter 4 focuses specifically on how abstinence was evaluated in terms of Ugandan frameworks for health and healing. It explores how abstinence was a practice driven by forms of spirituality and experiences of embodiment that diverged from Euro-American and biomedical orientations to health. I suggest that the ability to reframe abstinence in terms of these local orientations to spirituality and embodiment played a large part in how and why this became a popular health message within the Ugandan born-again community.

Chapter 5 examines the message of faithfulness as a prevention strategy and interprets how a message about planning for marriage was shaped by intergenerational conflicts in contemporary Kampala. I highlight especially how these conflicts played off young men's feelings of marginalization in the contemporary economy and how a message about AIDS prevention that asked them to withdraw from sexual relationships—usually a key measure of status for young men in Kampala—could succeed when paired with other neotraditional messages about gender relations and marital and household dynamics.

Part 3 begins with chapter 6, which serves as a coda for my ethnography of the church community as it focuses on the years after the end of the first phase of PEPFAR funding—a period when activism within the church expanded beyond AIDS prevention to address a wider array of concerns over sexual behavior. During this period members of UHC emerged as key participants in the antihomosexuality movement in Uganda, a series of protests that culminated in 2009 with the introduction in parliament of a bill that would radically intensify criminal punishments for men and women identified as homosexuals. This chapter analyzes the controversy over Uganda's Anti-Homosexuality Bill as part of the longer struggle to manage sexuality and gender relations in the late twentieth and early twenty-first centuries in Kampala.[59] In particular, it considers ideas about sexual personhood and sexual rights in Uganda today, and some of the problems faced by international and local groups that seek to protect gay Ugandans by building on rights-based arguments for sexual equality. Chapter 6 provides a window on how social activism within the church has changed in light of changing relationships with American Christians and a somewhat transformed political climate in the United States. Exploring the implications of accountability within other humanitarian endeavors, this chapter contributes a discussion of how efforts to extend the platform of human rights to include sexual minorities in Uganda has engaged and broadened many of the moral dilemmas I articulate earlier in the book.

Finally, this book's epilogue revisits the concept of accountability as a key framework for global health projects. In the years following the end of PEPFAR's initial grant period (2003–8), when abstinence and faithfulness fell out of favor as a dominant prevention strategy adopted by the U.S. government, members of UHC reflected on their role in a global AIDS prevention project. Their sense of frustration at the changing priorities of foreign funders revealed some of the limitations of global health partnerships that supposedly emphasize individual empowerment and personal accountability without acknowledging the ways that cultural, moral, and structural factors contribute to a community's experience of health and well-being.

PART I

❖

The Context of a Policy

1 AMERICAN COMPASSION AND THE POLITICS OF AIDS PREVENTION IN UGANDA

When President George W. Bush introduced the President's Emergency Plan for AIDS Relief (PEPFAR) in his 2003 State of the Union address it was remarkable for many reasons, but most notable was the dramatic shift it represented in the U.S. government's stance toward HIV/AIDS. It was not until 1986, a full five years after health officials began to track the spread of the epidemic in the United States, that President Ronald Reagan publicly uttered the term *AIDS* for the first time.[1] His long silence, a veritable erasure of the epidemic from official concerns during his first term in office, reflected a broader attitude of fear and indifference that permeated the Reagan administration's response to the rapidly unfolding health crisis.[2] Federal financing for AIDS-related research was also severely limited early on, in large part because of the opposition of prominent conservative politicians in Congress. Senator Jesse Helms, one of the most vocal of these opponents, gained notoriety for his declarations that the disease was the result of "deliberate, disgusting" conduct and thus was undeserving of scientific attention.[3] In the 1995 congressional debate over the reauthorization of the 1990 Ryan White Act, one of the first American policies that sought to secure care and treatment for Americans living with HIV/AIDS, Helms argued against refunding it. He told a reporter for the *New York Times* that "we've got to have some common sense about a disease transmitted by people deliberately engaging in unnatural acts."[4] Helms and his peers espoused the view that those who were dying of AIDS had behaved irresponsibly, even sinfully, and that these moral indiscretions made them accountable for their pain.

Given this, it is striking that less than a decade later President Bush, himself a conservative Republican, announced a global program to combat HIV/AIDS that is considered by many to be one of the largest and most important public health policies ever deployed. In his 2003 State of the Union address, Bush movingly argued that government policies are, at their best, vehicles for the personal compassion and care that Americans demonstrate to those in need everyday. Describing South African AIDS patients dying without access to treatment, Bush argued that PEPFAR represented a "work of mercy" capable of transforming the lives of millions suffering around the world.[5] With the stroke of his pen, AIDS moved from the margins to the forefront of U.S. health and global agendas. Even more remarkably, the AIDS patient was transfigured from the deserving sinner of 1980s urban America to the suffering victim (often in Africa, and often a woman) whose image seems so irrevocably linked to the epidemic today. What had precipitated this apparent about-face in how American conservatives viewed HIV/AIDS?

This question shadowed the early stage of my research in Uganda. In interviews I conducted in July 2004 with American and Canadian missionaries living in Kampala, the impact of PEPFAR was already evident. Members of Christian organizations that until that year had had limited involvement in HIV/AIDS treatment and prevention programs spoke to me in moving terms about their plans to become engaged with the issue and seek PEPFAR funds.[6] One middle-aged Canadian man told me how he had recently been "called" to the issue of HIV/AIDS and was expanding his mission's programs to address the epidemic. But the embrace of the issue was not without some conflict. Another missionary, someone who had dedicated most of his adult life to Ugandan relief work, confessed that until that year he had been little involved in AIDS programming, in large part because the U.S. churches that supported his work did not consider the issue to be central to a Christian mission like his. He explained that because HIV/AIDS was associated with "immoral behavior" it was difficult to find funding from religious American donors for such programs. Another missionary couple, who coordinated an AIDS education program funded by USAID, told me that they had prayed for a year, seeking to overcome their conflicting feelings about AIDS, before taking on the project. These views were not particularly uncommon. As Christine Gardner recounts in her study of U.S. sexual abstinence programs, a donor survey conducted in 2000 by the international Christian nongovernmental organization World Vision—just three years before Bush introduced PEPFAR—revealed widespread resistance among Christians to funding HIV/AIDS programs in Africa—even those serving orphaned children. One problem that World Vision leaders identified was the perception that AIDS sufferers "deserved their fate."[7]

For many of the Christian aid workers I spoke with that summer, the ground shift that precipitated their involvement in AIDS programming was related to changes in the ways AIDS patients themselves were perceived. No longer viewed as victims of their own misguided behavior, people suffering from AIDS—especially in places like Uganda—were seen as deserving candidates for compassionate intervention and aid. The introduction of PEPFAR, with its stipulations reserving a percentage of prevention funding for "behavior change" programs, bolstered the perception that AIDS prevention work could be a platform for social transformation and moral intervention. Moreover, Bush's faith-based policy initiative, which he had introduced in 2001, allowed for the broader engagement and direct federal funding of religious organizations in both domestic and foreign humanitarian and development work.[8] The couple above who were in the process of implementing their AIDS education program pointed to the faith-based policy as the reason they had taken on that project. The woman told me that "the U.S. [federal government] would fund our programs in the past—relief work and the like—but this AIDS curriculum development program? No way." Her implication was that the federal government had long considered most nonemergency humanitarian work done by missionaries to be outside the legal parameters of federal funding guidelines, which prohibit the support of projects that have a primary focus on religious proselytizing.[9] But now, under President Bush, religious and community organizations had been broadly encouraged to compete for federal funding and to occupy a more central role in the administration of a wide range of social services. On the ground in 2004 it seemed that PEPFAR and related U.S. federal policies were transforming the ways North American religious organizations considered the scope and impact of charitable and humanitarian intervention in Uganda.

In this chapter, I trace the significance of these shifts in attitude and engagement by considering the emergence and effects of an ethic of compassion within U.S. political discourse, an ethic that under President Bush's leadership came to shape how and why social welfare and international aid programs—and especially AIDS prevention programs—were pursued. My focus on compassion is an effort to analyze the underlying rationales that gave rise to PEPFAR in the early years of the twenty-first century, as well as the effects—intended and unintended—that followed the policy's implementation. My primary focus in the first half of this chapter is on American moral sentiments and ambitions: what drove American contributions to HIV/AIDS relief and prevention in Africa, and what forms did such contributions take?

My second aim is to explore the immediate effects of American compassion on the tenor of AIDS activism and on the landscape of AIDS prevention in Uganda. How was the American approach different from others that had—famously and successfully—preceded it? And, perhaps more significantly, what forms of social action and approaches to health and wellness did American compassion, with its ensuing emphasis on personal accountability, help generate?

America's Armies of Compassion: Making the Accountable Subject

President Bush's decision to address the global HIV/AIDS epidemic grew out of his efforts to develop what is now widely described as his "compassionate conservative" approach to governance. In the 2003 State of the Union address, Bush explained why he believed compassion should play a fundamental role in government policy. "Our fourth goal," he noted, "is to apply the compassion of America to the deepest problems of America. For so many in our country—the homeless, and the fatherless, the addicted—the need is great. Yet there is power—wonder-working power—in the goodness and idealism and faith of the American people. Americans are doing the work of compassion every day: visiting prisoners, providing shelter for battered women, bringing companionship to lonely seniors. These good works deserve our praise, they deserve our personal support and, when appropriate, they deserve the assistance of the federal government."[10] In the context of a federal policy speech, "compassion" invokes an ideal of the benevolent state, a government that identifies need and suffering and acts to address it. Yet Bush's compassionate conservativism sees compassion not as a value that the state itself possesses but one provided by its citizens.[11] It is a policy goal that seeks to pave the way for the empowerment of the private sector and private individuals who may address need and show compassion in their everyday lives, theoretically reviving a sense of civic responsibility and restoring the balance of moral governance in American society. Bush famously referred to charities and religious groups as "armies of compassion," better equipped than the state to address social problems like homelessness and poverty.[12] This was a compassion effected through the nurturing of a relationship not between the state and its needy citizens but between the state and a private sector sanctioned to serve the needy—battered women and lonely seniors—in ways believed to be more efficient and effective than those undertaken by the government itself.

This shift underscores how Bush's interpretation of compassion was marked by a broader inflection of neoliberal principles in his approach to governance and international aid. In the wake of 1990s domestic welfare reforms, individuals and the private sector were encouraged to participate in work previously relegated to the state and in turn were made more responsible for their own and their community's well-being.[13] The state's role in social programs was criticized by conservative backers of such reforms as inefficient, lumbering, and part of a legacy of progressive Democratic approaches to the problems of poverty that had supposedly created a relationship of dependency, rather than accountability, between citizens and the state. In the 1990s public policy rhetoric in the United States increasingly emphasized qualities like personal empowerment, self-esteem, and individual responsibility as the end products of a new free-market-dominated system characterized by looser labor regulations and a global corporate system hinged to a post-Fordist strategy of "flexible capital accumulation."[14] In the wake of these reforms, Bush's "compassionate" turn injected the image of the caring state back into the public consciousness. Yet the language of compassion, like these earlier policy endeavors, transferred the onus and responsibility of social services onto the citizen-volunteer, who was emboldened to take charge of social problems in lieu of state services.

The rise of a volunteerism as an expression of civic duty and as a key element of the transformation of the late capitalist state has been well documented.[15] President George H. W. Bush's famous "thousand points of light" speech, made at the 1988 Republican National Convention, presaged the celebration of volunteerism as an essential aspect of new forms of citizenship and social action that would come later. The Big Society program of British prime minister David Cameron provides a more contemporary corollary for how volunteer organizations have been heralded as essential tools through which society may compensate for the reduction of social welfare programs. Andrea Muehlebach's analysis of an emergent "moral" form of citizenship at the heart of the northern Italian neoliberal state has highlighted some of the key contradictions behind these trends;[16] her study of voluntarism in and around Milan from 2003 to 2005 notes how the heightened political emphasis placed on volunteer organizations during this period was driven by the desire to create a new "species of citizen" whose unpaid charitable productivity would fill the gaps created by a retreating postwelfare state.[17] Yet, contrary to a purely critical analysis, Muehlebach argues that the effect of this trend has been to complicate depictions of the neoliberal state as purely a rationalizing, amoral project. Similar to American conservative discourse, Italian reformers emphasize the emotional social bonds that are enhanced through volunteer labor; citizens are encouraged in Milan to "live with the heart," the message being that personal sentiment may animate state policy and make it more effective.[18] In this way the rise of volunteerism in Italy has been embraced by formerly critical sectors of society—such as the Communist Party and labor unions—for the ways in which such reforms are believed to generate new forms of "solidarity."

A notable aspect of this shift from state welfare to volunteer labor in both Italy and the United States is the way that services once considered to be the right of citizenship are encountered in this new version as a privilege, a "gift"—albeit ideally an emotionally resonate one, the product of a fraternal sentiment between citizen-donor and recipient. Marcel Mauss, in the conclusion to his famous essay on the gift, highlights connections between the emergent welfare state in early twentieth-century France and the reciprocal moral obligations that he views as emblematic of gift exchange.[19] In his idealized description, the interconnections among labor unions, workers, employers, and the state create a web of obligations that ensures security and solidarity for all. But in its late twentieth-century iterations the "gift" of compassion becomes both highly personalized and one-directional. The emphasis on volunteerism reimagines the gift of social services as unrequited, a demonstration of care in the face of abject need, seemingly given without expectation of compensation or reward. As much as the language of compassion sought to empower and mobilize American and European volunteers, it also undermined the agency of those who received aid. The needy were not partners in such works of compassion, viewed as members of a broader interdependent society, but instead were characterized as recipients of their neighbors' benevolence and care. The "right" to health care, safe housing, and food is reinterpreted in conservative language as a problem of "entitlements," a system that emphasizes the dependency, rather than the productivity, of the poor.

The context of international aid shifts the dynamic of the relationship of citizen and state to one of donor and recipient, but many of the effects of this rhetorical turn remain. The idea of compassion may be contextualized as part of the broader emergence in recent years of a "politics of care" that has shaped contemporary responses to humanitarian crises worldwide.[20] Erica James describes the "political economy of trauma" in Haiti as a "compassion economy," one that "can transform pain and suffering into something productive."[21] As Miriam Ticktin points out in her study of French asylum policies, the emergence of care as a platform for governance has shaped the subjects of the state's concern in particular ways.[22] The compassionate response is provoked by images of suffering, the recognition of a "morally legitimate" subject whose abject physical need compels our action. Drawing on Michel Foucault's notion of "biopower," a term he coined to explain the mechanisms through which life becomes the object of the state's "explicit calculation," Ticktin, James, and others have highlighted how the suffering body has emerged in recent years as the dominant platform upon which claims to state and nonstate resources may be made—a platform that has in many instances displaced and closed off other possibilities for collective political action.[23] This trend has perhaps been nowhere more evident than in the realm of international AIDS relief, where the ability to convey abject suffering to nongovernmental agents with the power to provide access to scarce medical resources may mean the difference between life and death.[24]

This recent work has brought about a question: When care or compassion becomes the central focus of international governance, what forms of subjectivity and political advocacy gain leverage? In the wake of policy reforms like PEPFAR, which infused major American global aid programs with the ethic of compassion and mercy, this question took a new shape: What kinds of "healthy" subjects and behaviors were made recognizable by the language of compassion, and why? Moreover, what effect did an emphasis on compassion have on long-standing and successful local efforts to prevent the spread of HIV in Uganda?

For President Bush and his advisers, the compassionate response was driven not only by the recognition of the suffering of others but also by the effect compassion itself was believed to engender. Bush described the compassionate approach as "outcome based, driven by results" and called for "compassionate results, not compassionate intentions."[25] He wrote in his administration's Armies of Compassion policy overview that "government should help the needy achieve independence and personal responsibility."[26] Compassion was viewed as a gift of redemption, a personal sentiment that when deployed enabled the social transformation of needy communities and individuals into accountable, responsible—but not "entitled"—persons.

These ideas were informed not only by a neoliberal orientation to governance but also by a distinctly Christian understanding of the nature of compassionate sentiment. For American Christians, Bush's language resonated strongly with familiar lessons about charity and the transformational effects of what evangelical Christians call the "selfless love" that characterizes demonstrations of mercy for the poor and suffering. Evangelical and born-again Christians believe that compassion "invokes an ideal of empathetic, unconditional benevolence,"[27] the demonstration of care in a context in which it may be least expected. Compassionate acts are selfless gifts but, perhaps paradoxically, they also engender an expectation of evidence of the transformational power of God's love. As Omri Elisha has discussed in his study of American evangelicals in Tennessee, charitable compassion is dialectically linked to an ideal of "accountability," the expectation that recipients of care demonstrate or reflect godly virtue.[28] The gift of compassion is on the surface understood as an act of selfless mercy, but it is also a gift capable of radical change, affecting personal conduct and, by extension, the moral fabric of society. In the eyes of conservative Christians at the turn of the twenty-first century, domestic welfare programs were redeemed by their transformation into programs of individual and community charity that were driven by the personal sentiment of compassion. Compassion in this American context was believed to address the problems of state welfare not only because the state became more efficient but because compassion combined care with the unstated expectation of personal change among recipients. A sense of empathy generated such Christian compassion, as did the possibilities for self-transformation that such a worldly (and spiritual) gift was thought to enable. By applying compassion to his global political agenda Bush signaled a similar emphasis on the transformational power of humanitarian mercy.

The idea that compassion was a transformational gift, one that engendered accountability in needy recipients, was a powerful tool in enabling the American conservative embrace of AIDS relief work, and for Bush's evangelical base this idea suddenly brought popularity to AIDS as a cause. Compassion was a sentiment driven not only by moral obligation but also by the "moral ambitions" for social change that extended from American ideals of volunteer and humanitarian work.[29] This was an orientation to charity and donor aid that was shaped in particular by evangelical Christian notions of what a demonstration of compassion meant and what response it should invoke. As I noted above, compassion in this instance was embedded not only in an idea of ethical obligation to those suffering but also in the notion of the work God's love does for and on the suffering subject. In American endeavors to show mercy, there was a parallel expectation that subjects would become accountable and empowered in return.

The language of compassion placed the onus on recipients of aid to demonstrate the transformational effects of their care. In the case of PEPFAR, such demonstrations were closely linked to an expectation that disease risk could be self-managed. If subjects of aid became more accountable for their behavior, especially by exhibiting better self-control, the forward march of the AIDS epidemic could be stalled. The years preceding and following PEPFAR's introduction in 2004 saw the growing influence of the language of "behavior change," an exhortation that encompassed a number of conduct-related prevention strategies. It became a popular concept for the Bush administration because of the ways it seemed to reinforce the sentiment behind the shift toward compassionate accountability as a key aspect of governance. Behavior change was celebrated as a strategy that emphasized individuals' own power to control their exposure to disease risk; if they could change when and with whom they had sex, and if young people could delay sexual debuts, AIDS could, in theory, be prevented.

For the remainder of this chapter I turn to the debates that surrounded PEPFAR's initial funding by the U.S. Congress in 2003 and the introduction of it in 2004, tracing the emergence of *behavior change* as a comprehensive prevention strategy and the contested meanings attributed to the term. Of particular interest are the ways in which compassion and behavior change transformed how Ugandans addressed and responded to AIDS. By 2004, when PEPFAR was implemented, individual actors, rather than communities, were made responsible for managing their own AIDS risk. As I will discuss, this precipitated a remarkable shift in the shape of Ugandan small-scale grassroots activism. I turn first to the global context and to the debates surrounding the funding for AIDS prevention and treatment that preceded PEPFAR's introduction.

PEPFAR, and Global Response

At the 2004 International AIDS Conference in Bangkok, Thailand, President Bush's proposal to spend $15 billion on global AIDS programs garnered widespread attention; the program's scope was radical by any interpretation. As recently as 2001 Peter Piot, the executive director of the Joint United Nations Programme on HIV/AIDS (UNAIDS), had confronted the United Nations' special session on HIV/AIDS with dire statistics outlining the extent of the global epidemic and the anemic response that donor nations had demonstrated to date. Piot spoke of the "collective shame" that marked inaction on the part of the world's wealthy nations and their responsibility to the dying in poorer ones.[30] That year international attention had focused on the expansion of the Global Fund to Fight AIDS, Tuberculosis and Malaria, which UN secretary-general Kofi Annan publically supported with his own personal pledge of $100,000. The Bush administration responded with a pledge of $200 million to the fund, with the stipulation that the UN project focus attention on prevention of HIV infection rather than treatment of AIDS.[31]

Global access to treatment had been a controversial issue at the International AIDS Conference held in 2000 in Durban, South Africa. Beginning in 1995, multidrug treatment with antiretrovirals had been shown to adequately control the replication of the HIV virus in patients. Antiretroviral (ARV) therapy had radically altered AIDS treatment in the West, transforming the virus into a chronic health problem rather than a death sentence, but treatment was expensive and complicated, demanding regular medical supervision to manage the high occurrence of side effects and the ever-present risk of developing resistance to some or all of the first-line treatment drugs. Detractors asserted that it was simply too complicated and too costly to provide treatment to the millions of HIV-positive persons living in resource-poor countries; activists countered that poor people were wrongly perceived as unable to follow the complex regime that ARV treatment demanded. Others lambasted the pharmaceutical industry for resisting the inexpensive reproduction of ARV drugs in generic form, a tactic that had been adopted by Indian drug companies and successfully used by the Brazilian government to facilitate its national treatment program, which had begun in 1996.[32] Limited access to treatment in the late 1990s and early years of the twenty-first century created a dire landscape of AIDS care, with those living in Western nations mostly assured of a life living with AIDS and those in poorer countries condemned to death. Miriam Ticktin's study of French immigration policies and Vinh Kim Nguyen's study of HIV treatment clinics in West Africa during this period describe the effects of such stark inequalities.[33] Access to treatment—either through international migration or through a petition to receive the limited aid of a donor agency—necessitated a triage approach to care in which the scarcity of resources demanded that health care workers evaluate need and suffering and decide on those most deserving of help.

It was into this environment that President Bush introduced PEPFAR. In contrast to a scenario of limited resources, of UN officials chiding donor countries to make donations for AIDS relief in the hundreds of millions of dollars, PEPFAR represented an infusion of cash of unprecedented proportions, with the vast majority of that money earmarked for treatment. The initial program pledge of $15 billion was to be divided between fifteen nations identified by the Bush administration as most affected by the epidemic, a list that included Uganda and was heavily focused on nations in sub-Saharan Africa.[34] Four-fifths of the money was directed toward treatment, a sum that immediately transformed debates over ARV access. To give some sense of the size and scope of the initial program, in fiscal year 2002—the year before PEPFAR was initiated—the U.S. government spent a total of $287 million on AIDS relief in Africa. By fiscal year 2006 that budget (including funding from PEPFAR) had expanded to nearly $1.3 billion, a nearly fivefold increase.[35] PEPFAR has dramatically expanded funding for both treatment and prevention in Uganda; for fiscal year 2008, the program accounted for $283 million of the $388 million in Uganda's budget for AIDS prevention and treatment and provided more than 70 percent of the country's entire resources for HIV/AIDS treatment and prevention, far outpacing the contributions of the Ugandan government and the UN Global Fund, Uganda's second biggest contributor to HIV/AIDS programs.[36] By all accounts PEPFAR is a program that has redefined HIV/AIDS treatment and care worldwide.

Despite these transformational numbers, PEPFAR was not wholeheartedly embraced by the global AIDS care community. As was noted in this book's introduction, the most controversial aspect of PEPFAR was that the program reserved one-third of its prevention funding ($1 billion) for abstinence and faithfulness-only programs.[37] At the 2004 International AIDS Conference in Bangkok the structure of PEPFAR's prevention funding drew intense criticism. An editorial in the *Lancet* described the tense reception at the conference of President Bush's Global AIDS coordinator, Randall Tobias: "Tobias was distinctly ill at ease and, for a few moments as he left the podium under strong verbal attack, it appeared that he would withdraw from the lecture."[38] Criticism extended from questions about the president's motives and especially the clear focus that Bush and the program's terms had placed on the role of religion in the fight against AIDS.[39] The *Lancet* editorial recounts Bush's speech, in which he touted an ABC approach (abstain, be faithful, and—adding the qualification "when appropriate"—use condoms) as a "moral message" and placed special emphasis on the importance of youth abstinence as an approach that prevents HIV "every time."[40] Many in the world of AIDS prevention distrusted the focus on abstinence, especially as it sought to drive funding away from other programs (in particular, those of condom distribution) that were perceived as less aligned with the Bush administration's social agenda.[41]

A Ugandan Christian activist I knew recalled for me his experience at the 2004 Bangkok conference, where he participated in a panel that seemed to dramatize the tensions of the moment. He was only in his early twenties at the time, and this trip—which took him halfway around the world—was the first time he had ever been on an airplane or traveled outside eastern Africa. At the time he was, he admits, unfamiliar with the landscape of international AIDS activism; his experience with AIDS advocacy extended only to his role as youth leader at University Hill Church (UHC), a congregation near Makerere University in Kampala that advocated premarital sexual abstinence. He had been selected as a youth representative for Uganda at the conference and was slated to appear on a panel discussing the role of abstinence programs in HIV prevention. He described to me his initial realization that controversy surrounded HIV prevention methods, especially abstinence:

> At that point I wish I knew better. I was in my final year at the
> university. It was an international AIDS conference. I was in Bangkok,
> in Thailand. It was my first opportunity to fly. It was really great. One
> of the greatest things, as a leader, is your story of transformation. So
> I had my story, you know. This is what had happened, this is what
> changed . . . I made the decision to abstain, and I'm just living my life
> and going on. And so I go over and I was simply supposed to give my
> testimony. And some guys were like, "Abstinence is an illusion, it
> doesn't happen." The guy who spoke before me, Dr. Steven Sinding
> [who represented] Planned Parenthood,[42] and then a girl from India.
> And I was like, "Guys, am I an illusion? I made a decision to wait! And
> I've been waiting, and it helped me!" So this was really eye-opening
> for me. There were four people presenting, but 80 percent of the
> questions came to me. But I kept the story. Some guys came and
> said, "Thank you very much for sharing the story." Then I talked to
> [prominent American evangelical minister] Rick Warren's son, shared
> with him some personal things, kept him in prayer, and then we kind
> of kept in touch.

Andrew had been prepared to "testify" in a mode of speaking common to evangelical and born-again Christians the world over. Testimonies are narratives of personal transformation shepherded by faith. In Andrew's eyes his faith had helped him abstain from sex, which had enabled his transformation from a sinful youth to a principled young man. For him this was a positive story, one laced with allusions to his own aspirations and personal achievements: nearing completion of his college degree and planning for marriage. This was a message central to the teachings in Andrew's church—that abstinence could be a strategy of upward mobility and social achievement—and it was one now being sanctioned by the U.S.

government. Andrew and his peers' experience with abstinence is a topic I will return to at length in later chapters, but the story he tells here is about the controversy that surrounded abstinence, and the sense of division within the world of AIDS activism that PEPFAR had seemed to generate. Andrew had been dropped into a struggle over public health policy that was animated by a broader conflict rooted in the U.S. religious and political landscape. In Bangkok, the first major international AIDS conference following PEPFAR's introduction, an American conservative coalition had, to an uncertain reception, thrust itself into the world of AIDS research and programming. Andrew's offhand mention of Rick Warren highlights the way in which PEPFAR and abstinence had emerged as a key arena for this American struggle, and the ways in which American politics and American religion had come to have an impact in even seemingly remote African communities. In fact, these African communities were placed at the very center of these debates.

Harnessing the Story of Uganda's Success: Defining Behavior Change

It was also at the Bangkok conference that the Ugandan story of declining HIV prevalence rates took center stage, in large part because the Bush administration had cited the country as evidence for why abstinence and faithfulness-only programs had been earmarked for special funding. Ugandan president Yoweri Museveni was a featured speaker at the conference, and he delivered a wholesale celebration of individual responsibility and self-control as frontline defenses against the epidemic:

> Eighteen years ago, as we emerged from a two decades protracted peoples' war of liberation against the dictatorial regimes of [Idi] Amin and [Milton] Obote, Uganda was once again under the shroud of a devastating mysterious ailment called "Slim," later to be known as AIDS. Two decades of civil war, state mismanagement and inappropriate monetary policies had left the Ugandan economy and social infrastructure in tatters with extreme levels of household poverty. The medical infrastructure, especially the hospitals, were in a sorry state with many of the medical profession living in exile, and the total per capita expenditure on health at less than $1 per annum. By 1985, Uganda was among the ten poorest countries in the world.
>
> We had to transmit to our people the conviction that behavior change and therefore control of the epidemic was an individual

responsibility and a patriotic duty and within their individual means.
In our fighting corner was a resilient population and a committed
leadership with years of fire-tested experience in mobilizing our
people to overcome obstacles at great odds and with minimal
resources.

Our only weapon at the time [was] the message: "Abstain from
sex or delay having sex if you are young and not married, Be faithful
to your sexual partner (zero grazing), after testing, or use a Condom
properly and consistently if you are going to move around. This has
now been globally popularized as the ABC strategy." With no medical
vaccine in sight, behavioral change had to be our social vaccine and
this was within our modest means.[43]

By the late 1990s, HIV/AIDS had become increasingly important to
Museveni's profile on the international scene, bolstering his image as a "new
African statesman" intent on supporting political reforms and terms for economic growth that were supported by his allies in the West. Uganda's government, like others across Africa, had become heavily dependent on foreign
donor aid during the 1980s and 1990s; by necessity Museveni had embraced
economic restructuring in 1987, opening Uganda to international donors who
had avoided the country under the Amin dictatorship of the 1970s, a period
that had been characterized by intense xenophobia and economic isolation
in Uganda. While Museveni had come to power in the mid-1980s as a leader
espousing "revolutionary" politics with an antielitist and broadly socialist
ideology of rural uplift, by the 1990s the locus of his power was clearly situ-
ated in and through the economic and political relationships he fostered with
the West.[44] The state's reliance on international aid expanded significantly
during the first two decades of his rule.[45] And, as was the case in other parts
of the world during this period, there were changes in the manner in which
that aid was distributed. The aid world had become radically decentralized
during the 1980s and 1990s, with direct state-to-state aid becoming a less popular model for donors.[46] Nongovernmental organizations (NGOs) and faith-
based organizations emerged as critical players in the local management
of donor funds.[47] These trends redefined the landscape of AIDS care and treatment in Uganda, a sector that has seen the expansion of medical research
projects fueled by donor funds.

Museveni's speech in Bangkok highlights many of these trends, especially
in the way he links economic restructuring to a successful HIV prevention

strategy he calls "behavioral change." In the years just prior to the Bangkok conference, *behavior change* emerged as a popular term highlighting individual accountability in health care choices. In Museveni's speech, avoiding disease risk by delaying sex and by promising faithfulness within monogamous relationships were celebrated as choices that buttressed other economic and political changes in Uganda. As Ugandans became more accountable, empowered, and self-reliant citizens, their nation supposedly also became more economically viable, more democratic, and better able to manage the epidemic that had ravaged its populace. In Museveni's words, control of the epidemic was an "individual responsibility" and within "individual means."

In fact, this language of self-sufficiency in many ways obscured the heavily community-based approach that Ugandans AIDS had embraced in the early years of the epidemic—strategies that emphasized accountability not only to one's self but to others, including those infected and at risk. Early prevention education emphasized peer-to-peer counseling rather than any top-down centralized curricula. Women's groups, newly empowered in the early years of the Museveni government, had organized themselves to address the impact of the epidemic on communities and families. But in a global context that emphasized neoliberal structural reforms, behavior change came to stand for liberal democratic ideals steeped in the rational, autonomous individual. One Ugandan public health student I interviewed in 2010 succinctly characterized the shifts from the 1980s to early years of the twenty-first century in Uganda when she said, "In the eighties there was a sense of communal vigilance [about HIV]. Communities became vigilant and aware of each other. It is not the case anymore. It is more about individual aid. [Prevention], now it's your call." By Museveni's calculation, behavior change seemed to represent these broader shifts in global sources of power and influence as well as the changing Ugandan economic and political context that marked early twenty-first-century life. Behavior change was a "technology of citizenship," to use Barbara Cruikshank's term, a mode of governance that has proliferated in the neoliberal era and "work[s] on and through the capacities of citizens to act on their own."[48]

What is most remarkable about the global adoption of behavior change is the way it came to replace earlier Ugandan strategies that focused more on community transformation than individual accountability. Long before there was widespread international focus on AIDS in Africa, Ugandans had in fact changed their behavior in ways that helped reduce HIV, but by the years of the new century the term *behavior change* had come to stand for something

American Compassion and the Politics of AIDS Prevention in Uganda

more particular than changing when and with whom one had sex. Perhaps more troublingly it was a term that obscured the broader structural shifts within Ugandan society that had made "changing behaviors" more feasible for many.

Uganda's "Miracle," and Sociostructural Components of Prevention

Rapid political changes emphasizing democratic participation and the increasing leverage of women and youth in local politics provided the critical backdrop to HIV programs of the 1980s and 1990s in Uganda. Contrary to his later incarnation as a Western-friendly advocate of open-market reforms, Museveni's early politics were influenced by his training at the University of Dar es Salaam in the late 1960s, a period defined by the expansion of Tanzanian president Julius Nyerere's *Ujamma* (African socialist) reforms. In publications during his first decade in power Museveni voiced an idealistic desire to politically mobilize the peasant classes in Uganda, and his early policies emphasized reforms of local government structures to encourage broad-based participation.[49] He has recently come under strong criticism for his long-held resistance to multiparty democracy (only retracted before the 2006 elections) and his iron grip on political leadership in Uganda,[50] but when he came to power in 1986 he was widely viewed as a political reformer who championed democratic governance and resisted corruption. The party leadership of Museveni's National Resistance Movement (NRM) opposed discrimination based on gender, age, education, and ethnicity.[51] Women and youth, traditionally groups with limited political influence, were given special consideration in electoral politics. Women's and youth seats were reserved at all levels of government, and in the first years of NRM rule women were far more successful in their campaigns for open parliamentary seats than they had ever been before.[52] Girls' enrollment in school also increased during this period, and the new Ugandan constitution, ratified in 1994, strengthened women's property and divorce rights.[53] The position of women significantly improved in the 1980s, and they responded to these opportunities by becoming more involved and organized at all levels of society. During this same period Ugandan villages became politically revitalized and a culture of local organizing to address community issues—encouraged by the NRM's grassroots politics—blossomed. Museveni's government also held a privileged position during these years, buoyed by widespread trust and optimism—both domestically and in the global sphere—for the possibilities of political change and the genuineness and transparency of government leadership.

It was in this context that initial efforts to address the impact of HIV/ AIDS emerged. Small rural communities in Uganda were faced with an almost unimaginably devastating epidemic in the 1980s, and the response within these communities was almost surely far more personal, small-scale, and community-centric than later efforts would be. The government and community messages surrounding HIV during this period were also clearly shaped by and responsive to local sexual attitudes. Museveni's famous "zero grazing" phrase, adopted by Bush administration officials as an example of a Ugandan message promoting abstinence, referred not directly to sexual abstinence but to a mere reduction in the number of sexual partners.[54] A comprehensive survey of Uganda's prevention efforts in the 1980s and early 1990s emphasized that no single behavioral shift can be credited with drops in HIV incidence during this period.[55] In a country where multiple concurrent partners are common, and where men view the support of multiple partners as a sign of their virility and status, many researchers argue that a message of no sex, particularly when levied at adults, would have fared poorly in these early years. Robert Thornton, an anthropologist who has studied Uganda's prevention success, quotes an army officer as saying, "Thank God, Museveni never told us not to have sex! He would have been laughed out of the country!"[56]

Ugandan organizations founded during the first decade of the epidemic, such as The AIDS Support Organisation (TASO) (which early on emphasized the social cost of the epidemic on women) and the youth education group Straight Talk Uganda were highly effective in using peers to educate about HIV/AIDS, encouraging open discussion of a previously taboo subject and disseminating information in a culturally sensitive manner. Peer-to-peer education has been shown to be particularly effective in making disease risk a personal matter and creating a stronger sense of social pressure to adhere to behavior changes.[57] Tellingly, Ugandans are more likely than any other Africans to have received information about HIV/AIDS from peers, as well as to have known someone personally living with the disease.[58]

In the 1980s and 1990s people in Uganda changed their behavior, delaying sexual debut and reducing their number of sexual partners. But such changes in behavior were also supported by significant structural shifts that had encouraged women and youth to take more active social and political roles in the country.[59] Moreover, the government supported an integrated, multisectoral approach to prevention that did not privilege any singular message or policy.[60] AIDS was a very real crisis; communities and the Museveni government responded by attempting to mobilize people against the disease, to talk about it candidly, and to use multiple approaches toward education and building awareness. Uganda's success was dependent on the individual actions of people who followed the ABC (abstain, be faithful, use condoms) message that became famous by the end of the 1990s, but such individual decisions depended in turn on a broader set of social and structural changes that involved communities in the response to the epidemic, worked to reduce the stigma of living with and speaking about AIDS, and encouraged women and youth to organize and address the different ways in which the epidemic affected certain groups.[61]

By the year 2000, the broader set of structural changes that had accompanied HIV prevention success were overshadowed by a narrowed focus on individual accountability and self-control as primary tactics of disease management. Behavior change reflected the rhetoric of the neoliberal reforms of this new era, privileging values like autonomy and self-sufficiency. Yet as I have briefly outlined here, a drive toward self-control had not always been the dominant message regarding HIV/AIDS in Uganda. As the nation's success circulated to the global level in the late 1990s, the story of its precipitous drop in HIV prevalence was applied as support for a broader U.S. political agenda that sought to emphasize the correlation between compassionate aid and the redemptive possibilities of personal accountability. Thornton recounts how USAID officials who had sponsored his research in an effort to prove that behavior change was the root of Uganda's success became dissatisfied when his work argued instead that abstinence had not been a key component of Uganda's early program.[62] By 2003, when PEPFAR was introduced, the narrative of Uganda's success had become contested terrain as various stakeholders sought to redefine why and how behaviors changed. This was nowhere more apparent than in the discussions that surrounded the initial funding of PEPFAR.

Ugandan Behaviors and U.S. Congressional Debates over PEPFAR

During the U.S. congressional debates that preceded PEPFAR's funding, Uganda's prevention strategy and the reasons for its success were strongly contested along political lines, with Republican lawmakers and Bush administration officials emphasizing the importance of abstinence and marital faithfulness to Uganda's ABC strategy and Democratic lawmakers resisting this characterization of Uganda's success. Testimony before the Senate and House subcommittees charged with addressing the new initiative demonstrated how Ugandan prevention policies were refracted through U.S. political and cultural divisions, leading to the program stipulations outlined in the 2003 legislation that funded PEPFAR. In one of the first of these meetings Representative Lois Capps, a Democrat from California, and Shepherd Smith, an American missionary with ties to the Bush administration, each framed Uganda's success quite differently.[63] Capps emphasized the integrated approach of Uganda's program and noted that abstinence alone had not been effective in Uganda, noting, "Reports from USAID and U.N. AIDS indicates [sic] that comprehensive and community-based approach to HIV/AIDS prevention works best. The fundamental goal of these public health interventions is to change behavior and it appears that Uganda's use of integrated behavioral change programs has had remarkable success. There is also no evidence that abstinence works alone. There is no data that sufficiently reports abstinence only rhetoric as causally decreasing rates of HIV/AIDS in Africa."[64] Smith—who, with his wife Anita, had founded a Christian NGO in Uganda—directly responded to Capps's comments, challenging her emphasis on an "integrated behavioral change" strategy: "I think that it's important to remember that this isn't ABC in the context that we think of comprehensive sex here in America. It's very targeted. It's abstinence to kids. It's be faithful to those in marriage or in monogamous relationships and it is [condoms] to very targeted communities such as the bars and the prostitutes and so on. So it is ABC, but it's not all lumped together. It's very segmented, [myself] having been there and looked at it very carefully."[65] In the years before PEPFAR, Ugandan AIDS programs were to a certain extent targeted toward certain populations and goals; many of these programs were developed and coordinated at local levels to address particular community concerns. But the sort of fracturing and policing of boundaries that Smith mentioned only became evident in the wake of PEPFAR's implementation; for example, it was in 2004 that Museveni removed any mention of condoms from school sex-education curricula.[66] As I discuss in the following section, in the wake of PEPFAR, U.S. efforts to categorize programs in order to evaluate them for funding established a new emphasis on the boundaries between distinct program areas, such as "condoms and related activities" and "abstinence/be faithful."[67] Smith's statements foreshadowed, rather than reflected, what was to become a much more fractured approach to AIDS care in Uganda.

Representatives of the Bush administration brought up Ugandan "culture" as justification for the abstinence and faithfulness focus of PEPFAR, often in surprising ways. Dr. Anne Peterson, the director for global health at USAID in 2003 and, by her own account, a former "missionary doctor in Africa," noted in testimony that "being faithful [to one partner] is a strong cultural norm that resonated strongly in Uganda and, from my own experience, I know it resonates also in many other African countries."[68] Many Ugandans would question this evaluation of Ugandan cultural norms or at least seek clarification of what "faithfulness" meant in the context of Peterson's speech. Long-term concurrent sexual partnerships (maintaining more than one regular sexual partner at one time) have in fact figured prominently in epidemiological explanations for Uganda's high HIV prevalence rates.[69] Peterson's comment also downplays the important distinction between Uganda's locally developed programs—the most famous of which, "zero grazing," targeted a reduction in the number of sexual partners—and PEPFAR's faithfulness message. The terms used during the congressional debates highlighted the difficultly of transposing and translating program guidelines cross-culturally. And in several cases they revealed surprisingly superficial characterizations of Ugandan culture and sexuality, rarely emphasizing the historical and social complexity of AIDS prevention in the country.

Most depictions of Uganda's program in the congressional record rightly focus on the issue of behavior change, but too often, as in the exchange between Capps and Smith, the debate came down to how important abstinence and faithfulness alone had been to Uganda's success. Uganda's far more nuanced and dynamic ABC program—integrating a variety of culturally relevant messages and dependent upon broader political and structural transformations—was lost in these discussions.[70] In Republican testimony, behavior change came to be limited to two specific behaviors—being faithful and abstaining—that were familiar and appealing to conservatives in the United States but that on their own failed to encompass the broader set of strategies and social and political shifts that had enabled successes in HIV prevention in Uganda. Behavior change came to represent personal responsibility for one's self, a discussion that was infused with references to Ugandan "tradition" and thinly veiled acknowledgment of Uganda's conservative religious and political environment.

In the debates over PEPFAR, Uganda's program was made the fodder for a particularly American political struggle—though one with global implications. Even so, this was not a battleground from which Ugandans were disengaged. American politicians sought out information about the Ugandan program in preparation to draft their own, and Ugandan First Lady Janet Museveni even traveled to Washington, DC in 2003 to help Republicans lobby for the dedicated abstinence funds in the PEPFAR legislation.[71] By 2003, several high-level Ugandan government officials publically supported an

THE CONTEXT OF A POLICY

emphasis on abstinence, especially for programs targeted to teenagers and schoolchildren. Janet Museveni, a convert to born-again Christianity, made the abstinence message a cornerstone of her agenda, spearheading youth abstinence programs through her office and, on World AIDS Day 2004, advocating a "virgin census" to encourage youth to remain chaste.

President Museveni and the First Lady were quoted in testimony during the U.S. congressional PEPFAR debates espousing a strongly proabstinence stance regarding sexual behavior in Uganda, with frequent references to the importance of self-control in the prevention of HIV infection.[72] This was not in itself surprising or new; there had always been competing claims to moral authority in the debates over HIV/AIDS in Uganda. Male elders claimed "tradition" as a bulwark against shifting gender and generational relations that they viewed as the cause of the epidemic. Women also claimed authority from their positions as caregivers and mothers that bolstered their attempts at organizing to prevent the spread of the disease. Museveni, as the country's most prominent political leader, would particularly be expected to chastise his population into behaving better. But PEPFAR's funding stipulations asserted a moral discourse that was not rooted in Ugandan notions of proper gender and generational relations or ideas about political patronage and obligation. The rising influence of an American moral discourse rooted in a U.S. Christian conservativism reoriented Ugandan struggles from local relationships to global ones.

Accountable Subjects: A Policy in Action

With the implementation of PEPFAR in Uganda, new political and social capital was gained by cultivating connections with organizations and funding sources abroad. These connections often depended on a facility for engaging with American conservative agendas privileging accountability and personal responsibility. Perhaps most devastating for Uganda was the way in which behavior change was set in opposition to other approaches to HIV/AIDS prevention. In the wake of PEPFAR, Uganda's broadly inclusive approach to program development was strongly challenged. Christians involved in prevention often told me that they wanted to change the meaning of Uganda's ABC prevention plan from "abstain, be faithful, and use condoms" to "abstain, be faithful, and lead a Christian lifestyle," seeking Christianity's prominence in and dominance over disease prevention efforts.

The immediate effects of PEPFAR were felt most keenly among NGOs who sought to apply for program funds. Uganda's prevention approach became more heavily fractured after PEPFAR's implementation, with organizations forced to account for how their programs supported specific PEPFAR funding areas. Sometimes a program's content had to be changed in order to satisfy these requirements. The prominent youth-focused group Straight Talk Uganda removed discussions about condom use from its educational radio shows after the American organization distributing PEPFAR funds to the group insisted that it do so.[73] The founder of that organization, a British national who has lived in East Africa since the mid-1980s, told me how the environment surrounding prevention work became more politically tense in the years following PEPFAR's implementation. The message of abstinence also became, in her words, "more rigid" and was increasingly informed by a Western view that understood sex to be driven by "only two things: desire and love." Programs that addressed the broader cultural context that informed decisions about sexuality in Uganda (for instance, Uganda's zero grazing program) were replaced by others better adapted to American grant requirements.

In order to seek PEPFAR funds, groups had to categorize themselves as addressing singular program areas, such as "abstinence/be faithful" or "condoms and related activities," that did not necessarily reflect the ways Ugandans had previously imagined and categorized prevention strategies. These classifications left little room for the more nuanced partner reduction messages that the Ugandan ABC program had been known for. Public perception of PEPFAR in Uganda was also that it heavily favored prevention programs focused on abstinence. In its report on the impact of PEPFAR in 2005, Human Rights Watch quoted one Ugandan youth: "With funding coming in now, for any youth activities, if you talk about abstinence in your proposal, you will get the money. Everybody knows that."[74] PEPFAR's own program report from 2005 also emphasized this focus, stating in the Uganda country section, "U.S. programming is increasingly emphasizing both A[bstinence] and B[e faithful]."[75]

The increase in donor funds for AIDS prevention also exacerbated the business-driven aspects of AIDS research and advocacy, in which a program's dependence on donor aid worked to reshape objectives to meet or synchronize with donor concerns. This was a problem not limited to AIDS funding, but its effects were keenly felt in the realm of Ugandan HIV/AIDS prevention. The director of Janet Museveni's Uganda Youth Forum, a youth-focused AIDS prevention NGO, articulated this dilemma when he told me in 2011 that, at the end of a grant's cycle, "You are left with unfinished business. But when the next resource comes you have either become irrelevant or they are focusing on another development area." PEPFAR represented a dramatic ramping up of both treatment and prevention programming, but it was marked by many of the problems that plague international aid in general. The terms of its funding were defined and driven by political agendas far removed from Ugandan communities. These agendas reshaped which messages were privileged and which became "irrelevant." Another long-term AIDS researcher in Uganda told me, "To me, the response to HIV/AIDS in Uganda was more effective before than it is now. Right now I see the overcommercialization—the overtechnicalization, and then the commercialization. People respond to money, not to the problem. The period before [now] there was no money. People were responding to the problem."

As international aid funding patterns have shifted, international NGOs devoted to HIV/AIDS prevention and treatment have become increasingly important social and economic institutions in Uganda. The effect of PEPFAR on Ugandan NGOs was perhaps most apparent in the rapid mobilization of Christian organizations, both local and international, that became involved in HIV/AIDS work. Large U.S.-based Christian NGOs played especially important roles in the implementation of PEPFAR; the largest grants under the 2003–8 program went to treatment projects (80 percent of PEPFAR's funds are dedicated to treatment), but international Christian NGOs, including World Vision and Samaritan's Purse, received significant grants for prevention.[76] Other smaller evangelical Christian NGOs, including some started by Ugandans, have also received funds. In 2007 Shepherd Smith, the missionary who testified before Congress, received a grant for abstinence and faithfulness programs on behalf of his NGO, the Children's AIDS Fund. His organization in turn relied on two Ugandan subpartners, Janet Museveni's Uganda Youth Forum and the Campus Alliance to Wipe Out AIDS, the latter founded by a Ugandan born-again pastor.[77] Both of these programs were dedicated to promoting an abstinence-only approach to youth education.[78]

These and other born-again organizations played a role in establishing the strong emphasis that Uganda's PEPFAR grantees have placed on abstinence and faithfulness as prevention strategies. In 2007, 39 percent of all of PEPFAR's primary grant recipients in Uganda listed abstinence and faithfulness as one of their program areas.[79] In 2008, PEPFAR's own statistics note that of 6.3 million Ugandans reached through prevention programs, more than 72 percent received an abstinence and/or faithfulness message.[80]

The emphasis on abstinence and faithfulness is not in itself radical in a country that for nearly fifteen years emphasized behavior modifications to reduce HIV prevalence. What changed dramatically under PEPFAR was how this message was being conveyed to the Ugandan population. Uganda's early program was thought to be so effective in part because it heavily relied on peer-to-peer education and locally produced content to educate about HIV prevention. The message about behavior risk was also integrated with other prevention messages, including partner reduction and condom use education, rather than viewed as a separate program area.

In Kampala in the years following PEPFAR's introduction the immediate sense was that AIDS prevention had become contentious and politicized in ways it had never been before. The experience of Straight Talk Uganda, whose program leader felt the group was on tenuous ground because its programs were not perceived as sufficiently proabstinence, gives only a partial picture. Prevention was a political issue, one shaped by international aid and Uganda's relationships with U.S. conservative lawmakers. In the years following PEPFAR's introduction, religiously infused prevention activism became a platform on which students and other young people could advocate for new attitudes about sex that were viewed as more aspirational, more empowering, and (from certain perspectives) more "moral." Troublingly, these messages were often placed in opposition to other prevention strategies that had previously been common in Uganda (the "zero grazing" program, or Straight Talk Uganda's long-form radio shows that emphasized peer-to-peer sexual education) as well as those approaches that most often contrasted with behavior change in global debates about prevention during this period (biomedical interventions such as serostatus testing and condom distribution).

A Fractured Landscape:
The Abstinence-Only Approach versus Condoms

At the 2006 World AIDS Day rally in downtown Kampala's Centenary Park the heightened tension between prevention strategies and advocacy groups was evident. Various HIV/AIDS treatment and prevention groups had gathered to celebrate their work in a leafy plaza off Jinja Road, a main downtown thoroughfare. Speakers took turns talking about the ongoing challenge of HIV/AIDS in Uganda. A group of students from UHC, one of the local churches active in promoting abstinence, were carrying banners and signs reading ABSTINENCE PRIDE and ABSTINENCE IS THE ONLY WAY OF PREVENTING AIDS that they had painted that morning at the church. During a presentation by another group, which mentioned its condom distribution program, members of the church group booed and shouted "Abstinence oye!" Throughout the rally any mention of the word condoms was met with a similar reception.

The apparent faultiness of other prevention methods was a fact often brought home by Christian abstinence activists in the years I lived in Uganda. A PEPFAR-funded student newspaper managed by a church-affiliated group on the university campus once ran a story explaining the "nine meticulous steps" involved in putting on a condom correctly. One young woman asked me, "If you can't be consistent with coursework, how can you expect to use condoms consistently?" Another pastor's presentation on youth sexuality in 2006 included a slide with a magnified sperm next to much smaller sexually transmitted viruses, the (misleading) lesson being that these diseases are so small they can permeate the latex in condoms. And a commonly repeated myth circulating among born-again Christian youth during a visit to Kampala in 2010 was that condoms cause cancer. This backlash against condom use was generated by the belief espoused by many Ugandan born-again activists, that abstinence (and, later, marital faithfulness) was the *only* way to prevent HIV/AIDS. In the years following PEPFAR's introduction the mobilization of religious actors and the increased funding for abstinence-only programs contributed to a growing environment of antagonism among HIV/AIDS groups in the country. Editorials in newspapers and speeches by politicians often offered support for one side of the abstinence argument or the other. The Church of Uganda, which had in earlier years demonstrated a relatively inclusive approach to prevention strategies (at times even counseling condom use), by this time had embraced a far more antagonistic stance regarding condoms. Church leaders adopted rhetoric condemning adultery and other "sexual sins" and promoted condom use only within marriage. Public rallies in central Kampala encouraged youth to consider abstinence the only way to prevent AIDS (see figure 1.1).

One of the most prominent church leaders to emerge during this period was Pastor Thomas Walusimbi, the founder of UHC, a congregation I will describe in greater detail in subsequent chapters. Pastor Walusimbi positions himself in Ugandan AIDS circles as a moral reformer, encouraging "appropriate" behavior as a way of preventing HIV/AIDS. He expertly emphasizes how abstinence and faithfulness are Ugandan cultural values that have been undermined by foreign AIDS agendas that he views as biased against a faith-based approach to HIV/AIDS prevention. During a speech on AIDS leadership given on the university campus in 2007 he characterized his work as a struggle against a foreign AIDS prevention establishment that is populated by experts who are "liberal, faithless, and have no families." His message appealed to conservative American Christians, who also saw themselves fighting a moral battle against a nonbelieving, liberal establishment, as well

51

American Compassion and the Politics of AIDS Prevention in Uganda

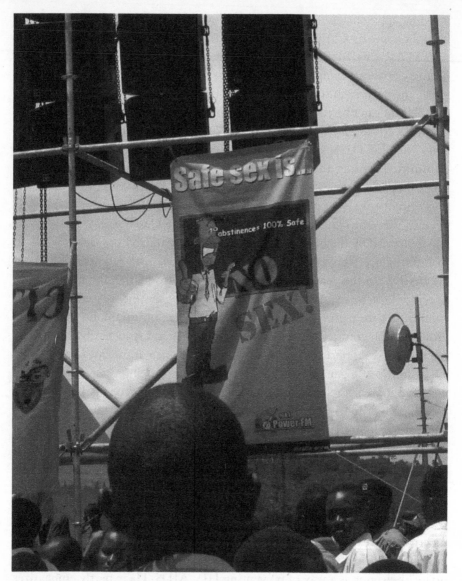

FIGURE 1.1. "Safe sex is no sex!" rally in support of abstinence, Kampala, October 2006

as to an African audience for whom calls for a reassertion of "traditional" African gender and family norms in response to the social disorder of HIV/ AIDS had become common. For young Ugandans, however, Walusimbi's narrative of resistance to the corrupt influence of seemingly amoral foreigners provided a message about their own self-empowerment and global influence

THE CONTEXT OF A POLICY

that was deeply appealing. When I interviewed him, Pastor Walusimbi elaborated on this argument, noting, "Africans have been so relegated to the backseat of development and modernism for so long. And there is a sense in which we always receive, we never give, we never create. Our stories are told for us. It really makes me weep. Even when we have a successful story, like our HIV/AIDS story is a successful story. Even then someone has to come and say this is what you did, this is how you brought HIV/AIDS down." Walusimbi claims that Uganda is not recognized for the success it had curbing HIV prevalence primarily because foreign HIV/AIDS policy makers resist talking about morality in the context of AIDS. Ugandans, he noted, are "religious, we're family oriented." Therefore, he argued, the people are responsive to a message of abstinence and faithfulness. As I have outlined above, the story of Uganda's success is far more complicated than Walusimbi would have it be. But the rhetoric he uses to couch his criticisms is attractive, emphasizing Ugandans' own moral authority and autonomy in the fight against AIDS—a fight that is now, undeniably, driven by a global economic and political agenda far removed from Ugandans' home communities.

While Walusimbi frames his protest against the perceived intrusion of external funders and their "amoral" agenda, his message gained prominence because of the worldwide controversies surrounding American HIV/AIDS policy. He characterizes his message as one of Ugandan youth empowerment, but the message's power is derived from a connection to international—and especially American—Christian discourses regarding morality and AIDS. The meaning Ugandans attribute to Walusimbi's message about personal accountability and self-control is an issue I take up in later chapters. But the landscape of AIDS activism in the early years of the twenty-first century, an era deeply shaped by a compassionate response on the part of President Bush's conservative religious base, can be followed in Walusimbi's rhetoric.

Conclusion

In the late 1980s and into the 1990s Ugandans did in fact adapt their behavior, delaying sexual debut and reducing their concurrent partnerships—effectively abstaining and becoming more faithful, thus reducing HIV prevalence in the country. But the story of PEPFAR is a story of how behavior change was taken out of the broader structural and cultural matrix that had brought it force and shape and how it was given a new kind of agency through the ideals of "compassionate care" championed by the U.S.

government. Starting in 2003, when *behavior change* was adopted as a buzz-word by President Bush and his advisers, abstinence and faithfulness had evolved into a singular abbreviation for individual choices that emphasized personal accountability for disease risk and prevention—choices that could be promoted and exported globally. This was an interpretation of prevention success that buttressed other objectives of American humanitarianism of the era, an orientation to compassionate aid that helped outline and reinforce the dominant frameworks of neoliberal social action—autonomy and individual agency—that often obscured alternative ethical practices and modes of action that had figured prominently in earlier Ugandan efforts to mobilize against the AIDS epidemic. In chapter 2, I take up the Ugandan context more directly, focusing on the history that lead up to the introduction of PEPFAR. This is a history not of the epidemic itself but of forms of moral activism in the face of social change, activism that informed the more recent iteration of moral authority so effectively claimed by Walusimbi and his peers.

2

AIDS AT HOME

Urbanization, Religious Change, and the Politics of the
Household in Twentieth- and Twenty-First-Century Uganda

In 2006, I attended a gospel music concert, organized by local churches to promote youth abstinence, at the upscale Serena Hotel in central Kampala. At the beginning of the concert a high-profile army colonel gave an introductory speech drawing surprising corollaries between AIDS and the ongoing war in northern Uganda.[1] The main emphasis of his speech was that both tragedies—the war and the epidemic—had been caused by an erosion of cultural values. Young people, he explained, had forgotten how to "behave." AIDS, he continued, was "not being helped by this business of boyfriend and girlfriend." He stressed that the norms of "traditional culture" dictated that marriages should be arranged by families, not according to the whims of young people's desires. His comments drew a frightening parallel between the horrors of the civil war and the sexual promiscuity he blamed for the epidemic: both were supposedly driven by a growing lack of civility and respect for cultural norms.

Within AIDS prevention circles, "culture" has become a touchstone in debates that have tried to sort out why some approaches to prevention succeed and others fail. Uganda's early AIDS education programs have been described as "culturally grounded" and in tune with the "nature of African society,"[2] qualities that set them in opposition to global biomedical or technological interventions that are less effective. As I discussed in chapter 1, American advocates of the President's Emergency Plan for AIDS Relief's (PEPFAR) emphasis on abstinence used references to "Ugandan culture" to defend PEPFAR against accusations that it was out of touch with the realities of the African AIDS epidemic. What these arguments usually fail to recognize are the ways that culture, especially so-called traditional culture, are contested ideas within affected communities themselves. As we can see in the speech by the colonel, for Ugandans the terms *culture* and *tradition* are often embedded in the rhetoric used to describe the epidemic's scope and proposals toward stemming its spread. Far from static concepts, references to cultural values provide a way for diverse groups of people to intervene in discussions about the virus and comment upon the social costs of changing attitudes toward gender, sexuality, and the family.

In the previous chapter I described how the post-PEPFAR embrace of accountability as a key element of prevention programs was shaped by the terms of an American debate over "compassionate" neoliberal reform and the moral worth of self-sufficiency and autonomy. In Uganda, *culture* and *tradition* were equally important concepts that animated the language of account-ability and spurred support for the message of abstinence and faithfulness. In contrast to the American celebration of compassionate aid, animated as it was by an investment in the redemptive worth of the autonomous subject, Ugandan debates surrounding abstinence and faithfulness were concerned with questions about the shape of moral obligations to others during a period of rapid social change: What kinds of families and persons are deemed proper and good? What is the social worth (and potential cost) of personal indepen-dence or monogamy? What kinds of marriages are moral and worth protect-ing? These were not questions sparked only by the crisis over the AIDS epidemic, or the contemporary climate surrounding neoliberal aid (though these events have made such questions more urgent); they were questions that drew on a century's worth of debates over the place of "traditional" culture within the modern state.

The present-day Ugandan Christian effort to find political capital in the defense of so-called traditional values is hardly a new strategy. As early as the first decades of colonial rule, reformers sought to address the perceived problems of urban life and colonial culture—sexual "deviancy," women's new "freedoms," the "loose" relations between young women and men—by as-serting the language of tradition as a safeguard against the social costs of change. Colonial processes of urbanization, and the dramatic changes to family and social life that followed, precipitated questions about the effects that an abandonment of "good manners" and cultural values could have. Responses to the AIDS epidemic, especially debates over the moral value of certain orientations to sexual and gendered behavior, have their roots in these colonial-era efforts—by British and Ugandan, traditionalist and Christian—to forward varied (and often contradictory) arguments about the social pur-pose of customary life in a changing world.

In the pages that follow I trace the emergence of a moral authority—rooted in efforts to reform the family and home, and articulated using the language of tradition—as a political force in colonial and postcolonial Uganda. The emergence of the home as a political project during the colonial era—one made palatable because it was formed on private, "moral" terms, and thus conveniently outside the scope of state politics—helped foster new forms of social protest over the terms of colonial rule. These were efforts to reimagine the political and intimate relationships of Ugandans—relationships that had until the colonial period been fundamental to ideas about health, well-being, and the nature of successful communities. This was an authority vested in individuals who sought to defend and reimagine norms of obligation, sociality, and behavior by making powerful claims about what traditional culture is and what it does.

This is a history that continues to inform the Ugandan Christian modes of political protest that have emerged since the first decade of the twenty-first century. More than replicas of their American religious counterparts, the Ugandan born-again Christian activists I describe in the following chapters are shaped by this particularly Ugandan history and speak on terms that relate to Ugandan concerns about—and orientations to—moral community and personhood. If chapter 1 traced American Christian political involvement in AIDS prevention to the emergence of an ethic of "compassion" for the needy, the present chapter will trace the politicization of Ugandan Christians to the mobilization of the idea of the traditional home as a concept worth not only defending but also reforming. PEPFAR's ideal of the "accountable subject" was refracted through these long-standing debates that sought to define the moral worth of different forms of family life and intimate relationships in Uganda.

Two notable moments in the colonial history of the family and household mark important turns in the history of Christian social protest in Uganda and highlight how the reinterpretation and defense of "traditional" family life became a key platform for Christian politics in the twentieth and early twenty-first centuries. The first was the debate over marriage sparked by the expanding influence of Protestant Christianity in the British Protectorate of Uganda during the colonial era. The second was the advent of the East African Revival in the 1930s, a reaction to the dominance of an elite Protestantism in the early twentieth century that is notable for its emphasis on the public confession of sexual sin. These moments present nearly opposite reactions by Ugandans to changes in their society. The first controversy—concerning forms of marriage in the colonial state—revolved around arguments over the importance of extended kin relationships to people's lives. A prominent group of traditionalists argued that these relationships were necessary for morally sound families and marriages, and that to do away with the bridewealth ceremonies that emphasized such ties (a move encouraged by Western missionaries) posed a threat to social stability during a period of upheaval and change. The second controversy—the East African Revival—was one in which "traditional" forms of moral authority were eschewed in favor of new practices of personal asceticism. Revivalists encouraged moral reform of the self, especially as forged through public rituals of confession. To compare these historical periods demonstrates the ways in which "tradition" was a concept in flux throughout the colonial period and afterward. Both of these events, and the reactions to them, helped shape the ways that Ugandans think about ideal families and healthy sexuality today. The narratives that developed in response to these historical moments, narratives about family life and the moral purpose of marriage, are recognizable in and even central to the arguments presented by born-again Christians today in response to AIDS.

Transformations to Marriage in Buganda during the Early Colonial Period

Kampala lies at the center of the precolonial kingdom of Buganda, which at its largest extended east to the Nile River and north as far as the Kafu River (see map 2.1). In the late 1800s at the beginning of the colonial period, Buganda was the largest and most powerful of the precolonial interlacustrine kingdoms of the African Great Lakes region. It was an intensely hierarchical and bureaucratically sophisticated state, with regional chiefs (bakungu) appointed by the king (kabaka) to manage the far-reaching territories of the kingdom.

The history of Kampala is in large part a history of the Ganda people's efforts to corral and reimagine the place of their own customs within the colonial city and state. The household, as a moral barometer of change, was placed at the center of these struggles. Far from depoliticizing family life, colonial interest in the domestic sphere intensified the home's political and moral worth; the household emerged as a key locus of social change during the colonial period, inciting fierce debate among the Baganda about the long-term implications of alterations to the family, and concerns about family life became the focus of political critiques that sought to address the costs of these changing forms of power and authority.

In precolonial Buganda, marriage and family were understood as elements of larger networks of mutual support and obligation that provided access to land and the social and economic power that came with such access. As a site of material and social reproduction the household was viewed as a

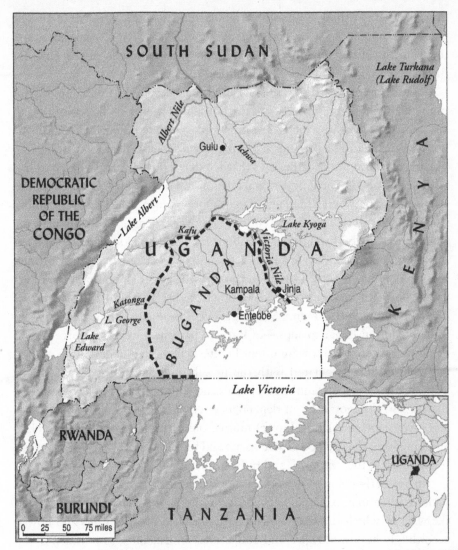

MAP 2.1. Uganda and Buganda

component of the precolonial state, governed by relationships of mutual obligation and reciprocity that were mirrored at the nexus of royal power. As much as it was an economic and political unit, the household was also the locus of moral reproduction, where modes of behavior and conduct were learned and cultivated. Derek Peterson has written that in precolonial East Africa "diverse peoples had long upheld different models of discipline, but everyone agreed that an honorable reputation was built at home."[3] In Buganda the household was where one was taught discretion, obedience, and the elements of respectability (*ekitiibwa*) and good manners (*empisa*) that defined proper conduct and enabled political success.[4]

One's clan provided the spiritual and bureaucratic roots of belonging for individuals and family groups, but the household itself was the moral, social, and economic unit to which most individuals oriented their lives and livelihoods. Buganda was a patrilineal and patrilocal society, meaning that descent was traced through the father and that women left their natal village to live in their husband's. The foundational relationship that formed a household was the marriage between a man and one or more women. Marriage was, and to some extent still is, a means to control and organize access to economic resources, especially through the distribution of land by older men to younger ones. The practice of bridewealth exchange necessitated that younger men acquire material wealth (usually in the form of livestock and other agricultural goods) in order to marry—a practice that required the support of older, more powerful men.[5] Marriages were moments when ties between individuals and larger groups—of kin and patrons—were reinforced. And bridewealth ceremonies were often the sites where such negotiations among various interests associated with the new household might play out. For both women and men, adulthood in Buganda might be said to have required the successful negotiation of dependence—that is, the proper management and investment in relationships of mutual obligation (of home, family, clan, and kingdom) that helped enable social and political success. Marriage was a relationship at the center of, and fully animated by, such efforts.

In the early colonial period the household became an object of intense social transformation, especially as land policies and marriage laws altered the ways in which the state viewed individuals and family units and how it accordingly bestowed rights and obligations. In Buganda, as in much of the rest of Africa, the colonial period introduced a new sense of separation between political and domestic power, relegating most elements of women's authority to the latter. Victorian understandings of gendered difference helped shape political and moral worlds as distinct realms. Women were repositories of society's moral virtue; men abandoned such virtue to excel in the political and market-oriented world, returning to the female-dominated domestic sphere to recover from the strains of their sinful ambitions. Men's status, long associated in part with the successful creation of a home in Buganda, was transformed into a new project of worldly achievement that necessitated the pursuit of educational degrees and wage labor. Colonial attitudes effectively transformed men's power by at least partially divorcing it from the marital and kin relationships that had long provided a route to political influence in Buganda and elsewhere in the protectorate.[6] Throughout Africa these changes affected women's social status in particular, as African political systems predicated on notions of gendered interdependence that viewed the domestic sphere as being integral to other forms of social and political authority went unrecognized by colonial rulers.[7] Women, whose relationships with men had helped articulate male power, became instead associated with a distinct domestic realm. Far from depoliticizing family life, however, colonial efforts to define and reform the domestic sphere were intense, and the household became a key locus of political and social change.

The reform of marriage was at the center of these transformations. The colonial state and foreign missionaries viewed marriage—particularly the regulation of a monogamous marriage ratified by an oath of mutual consent and authorized by both state and church—as a necessary part of the "civilizing" process. Marriage was viewed as an institution through which the colonial state might better manage African behavior and inculcate modern virtues. Such reforms were often enacted in the name of women's protection and with the notion that marriage could rein in men's and women's sexual appetites. During the early decades of the twentieth century, missionaries forged a decidedly antagonistic view of Ugandan cultures. Anglican missionaries engaged in efforts to effectively do away with many of the small-scale family ceremonies that were at the center of experiences of social reproduction and moral stability in precolonial Ganda society. Children's naming rites,[8] ceremonies celebrating the birth of twins,[9] and the kwabya lumbe "succession" ceremonies conducted after death were all attacked by church leaders for promoting a "magical" spirituality and inappropriate ideas about gender and sexual behavior,[10] but the church's foremost concern seemed to center on Ugandan marriage law. Throughout the early decades of the twentieth century, foreign missions repeatedly sought to reform colonial laws in order to ensure certain models for Christian families and to do away with customary marriage (especially bridewealth ceremonies), which they believed to be immoral and degrading to women.[11] Under the terms of Britain's "indirect" style of rule, where colonial law recognized both African customary and British common-law marriage statutes, missionary efforts focused throughout the first half of the twentieth century on reinforcing the superiority of Christian monogamy. In 1938 an Anglican missionary made clear his discomfort with the persistence of multiple pathways to marriage: "It is not the duty of government to make it easy for Africans to marry as they like, but to educate them up to the right conception of marriage."[12]

European missionaries viewed Christian monogamous marriage as a repository for a certain type of moral and gendered virtue that they believed to be integral to the modern world. In response to an Anglican Church survey that sought to elucidate the benefits of Christian marriage for Ugandans, one missionary wrote in 1931, "Those 'legally' married [in church] would have a strong deterrent from falling into loose ways and dishonoring their marriage vows. Christianity in Uganda still seems in its infant stage in which punishment is necessary, as well as teaching, for the building of character and formulation of right minded public opinion."[13] For both the church and the colonial state, marriage was understood to be at the center of the creation of a modern civil society; as an institution, monogamous state-sanctioned marriage emphasized ideas about the obligations and rights of citizenship and the behaviors associated with democratic free will. The church recognized marriages that had been sealed not by bridewealth exchange but by an oath of consent, the assertion ("I do") by two individual parties that stated their intent to marry.

Christian and state-sanctioned marriage introduced new ways of thinking of the self—as rights-bearing and autonomous—as well as new ways of thinking of one's relationships with others. People were taught to consider marriage a union between two "consenting" individuals rather than a relationship that joined two extended families and organized a broader set of kin-based relationships and obligations. This had implications for how people thought about the role of family life within the state and the nature of the moral authority that families were thought to extend.

Elite Baganda initially embraced Christianity and Christian monogamy as essential foundational steps in the process of building a "civilized" colonial leadership within the kingdom.[14] The equation of political and economic power with particular religious identities created a new politics of morality during the early twentieth century; elite Protestants sought to distinguish their way of life from those with less power and influence, and in many cases this involved embracing missionary arguments about what constituted proper family relationships and domestic ideals.[15] Far from resisting efforts to do away with polygamy and bridewealth, the landowning elites at the top of the Ugandan colonial hierarchy embraced monogamous church unions as symbols of their newfound wealth and status. One Ganda petitioner of this period went

THE CONTEXT OF A POLICY

so far as to argue that Africans should no longer be subject to the apparent incivility of customary polygamy; it was England's duty to "put into force the English law for the African Christians. Christianity is the ruling religion of England and the British Empire. Polygamy is next to Bolshevism."[16] Recognizing the powerful association of Christian marriage with status, one missionary commented, "Many progressive Africans would favour the recognition of monogamy by native law, if only from a desire to emulate more civilized social institutions."[17]

By the beginning of the twentieth century Buganda had seen a radical reform of the idea of marriage, at least as it was celebrated by urban elites. Christian marriage became a marker of status in the kingdom, one that was not only symbolically but also politically and economically transformative. These new marriages were aligned with European ideas about personal ownership, individual rights, and a new orientation to the state that viewed the domestic sphere as a realm set apart. The importance of the extended family, clan, and patronage relationships that had been the basis for leaders' moral authority and political legitimacy in precolonial Buganda seemed to recede. But the power of this new Christian elite was soon met with resistance that was formed using language that questioned the moral costs of such intimate transformations.

A More Moral Progress? The Bataka Union and the Resurgence of Custom

In the 1920s a pervading sense of "moral crisis" colored public discussion of the social changes that had followed from colonial rule—especially the perception that elite Christian chiefs had misused their new power and wealth.[18] The Bataka Union emerged as the "common" man's response to this crisis, and it was a response that was deeply critical of the power that had been consolidated by Christian Ganda chiefs at the expense of ordinary citizens. *Bataka* referred to the name used for the clan leaders who had managed ancestral claims to land in precolonial Buganda. The use of this term emphasized the grounds for the new group's complaint; its members drew on the language of "tradition," demanding the protection of customary and ancestral claims to land by peasants and clan leaders—claims that had been superseded by a new elite politics oriented toward the church and colonial state. As "spokesmen for authentic culture" this group also advocated for "stronger" marriages and spoke out against what were characterized as new instances of "sexual prolificacy" and the spread of sexually transmitted diseases.[19] The

Bataka Union criticized Ganda leaders for embracing sexual deviancy and excess and advocated for a return to customs that they believed preserved traditional moral norms, such as female virginity and fidelity within marriage.[20]

Their criticisms pointed to the ways colonial-era political rebuke was increasingly framed in terms of sexuality and intimate behavior. The greed of Buganda's Protestant leaders was equated with sexual degeneracy in the society at large. The new forms of sexual "excess" that petitioners complained about were linked to the social costs of new forms of elite power. This is not surprising given how political power had been conceived prior to colonial rule: precolonial leaders had been considered responsible to and for their followers, and political rule had been viewed in part as a personal, intimate relationship. Emphasizing this, Holly Hanson has even described political authority in Buganda as a relationship conceived in terms of "love and affection."[21]

Bataka critics attempted to use this moral language in new ways. Powerful men had long been able to assert degrees of sexual excess in their lives,[22] and polygamy had previously been a key way that political authority and status were both created and publicly demonstrated.[23] Thus, Bataka criticisms of new leaders' "sexual prolificacy" pointed to a shift: the moral breakdown of society, of relationships between leaders and subjects, was translated by the movement into other forms of moral misbehavior—specifically a sexual "misbehavior" that had previously been overlooked, and even encouraged, in powerful men. Sexual behavior emerged as a primary way of talking about the problems of power and the breakdown of social norms.

If Bataka Union members sought to expose the moral costs of new forms of leadership, they also shifted what it meant to pursue a "traditional" family. Theirs was an argument that viewed "traditional" values themselves—and not the Christian church or new forms of state control—as the safeguards against what was viewed as the moral threat of new forms of political and economic power. Yet the practice of monogamy, and not customary polygamy, became their ideal marital status, one that they argued reinforced traditional values like personal restraint and self-control. Thus, even as tradition was reasserted as an important aspect of colonial life, ideas about what constituted a "traditional" marriage, and traditional sexual morality, were changing.

Bridewealth ceremonies became an especially important part of these arguments. If Bataka reformers espoused the benefits of monogamy, they also defended the moral worth of traditional bridewealth exchange to seal such unions. Missionaries had long asserted that the practice of bridewealth exchange reduced marriage to a material exchange that undermined the sanctity of the individual. But by the 1920s Baganda traditionalists were arguing that, to the contrary, Christian unions were what led to a devaluation of marriage, enabling young people to enter rashly into a partnership without any of the social support and deeper moral meaning inferred through bridewealth exchange. A Christian marriage without bridewealth was a marriage with no foundation or sense of social rootedness, they argued. A marriage of individuals was a weak union; a marriage conferred through bridewealth was a more stable, more moral union, bound by the network of social relationships that had supported and enabled the marriage.

Here "traditional" culture is reimagined and given new terms and a new purpose. Rather than opposing modern progress, Bataka Union leaders sought to ground modern change—specifically, monogamous marriage—in the moral authority that was derived from traditional customs. Customs and Christianity were reframed as parallel, rather than antithetical, projects of collective morality that together enabled "forward progress."[24] This was a remarkable shift in rhetoric that both upheld Christian monogamy as a new, valuable model for marriage and asserted that it was only through the continued practice of bridewealth that such a monogamous marriage could withstand the threat of modern vices and remain a moral union. With these arguments the reform of marriage became the grounds for addressing political instability and the seemingly moral misbehavior of new leaders.

If the debates forwarded by the Bataka Union revealed the enduring importance of and transformations to the idea of "tradition" within the colonial state, they also emphasized the ways colonial criticisms of the changing nature of political authority were often expressed in terms of the "problems" of gender and sexuality. Jesumi Miti, one of the Bataka leaders, told the kabaka of the sins befalling his subjects because the kingdom no longer oversaw marriage and marital disputes: "to day women every woman moves the way she wants . . . because there are no longer the good morals that our great-grandparents had that still are there in Buganda today."[25] Miti came to celebrate customary bridewealth and sought to reassert the tradition of husbands confirming their wives' virgin status on the marital bed.[26] Chastity, virginity, and fidelity to one partner became rallying cries in response to perceptions of the social ills that many associated with changing social dynamics. Sexual and family problems came to symbolize the broader breakdown of the moral authority of the colonial state. Family life was viewed as a barometer of the costs of change, and interventions focused on both the reform and rehabilitation of marriage and the household.

There is no doubt that this revival of custom was attempted in the face of destabilizing social changes—especially changes to the urban landscape of

Kampala. By midcentury, women and men were likely to cohabit without marrying rather than pursue a church wedding or a bridewealth ceremony.[27] By the postwar period there were a range of domestic partnerships that exceeded the familiar dichotomy of customary versus Christian unions. Common partnerships included "free marriage," an unofficial long-term union between a man and woman that was informally but not legally recognized.[28] Resembling this domestic arrangement, but considered less respectable, were "lover" or "friend" (*mukwano*) relationships whereby a woman lived in a man's home and received gifts in exchange for domestic chores.[29] In most cases people in cities lived far removed from their families, surrounded by strangers. Lucy Mair wrote in a 1934 study of Ganda marriage that private land-ownership had made people more mobile, less bound by the ties of kinship that had previously afforded men access to land and livelihood. Women had also become more "independent," with greater access to a wage-based economy. Mair argued that these changes had made marriages less stable and households more prone to continual rearrangement. In her survey of fifty-eight households, only eleven were those of monogamous first marriages. She found nineteen single adult men and women living without a partner, a situation that would have been highly unusual and considered morally suspect in precolonial Buganda.[30] In the face of such transformations, efforts to reassert the language of tradition as a morally stabilizing force was an effort to preserve, and to a degree transform, certain ideas about the household and home, the place of the family at the center of a broader network of relationships many believed sustained moral and social health and well-being.

The East African Revival: Confession and Public Discussion of Sexual Sin

In light of these efforts to reassert a version of tradition into colonial life, the followers of the East African Revival were radicals, advocating a complete break from customs and a renewed embrace of Christian spirituality; the movement was critical of elite Christians and traditionalists alike. The revival began in 1929, in what is now Rwanda, and quickly spread into Uganda and much of the rest of eastern Africa. Revivalists were called *balokole* (saved ones) in Buganda, and were soon infamous for their subversive behavior: the disruption of church services, the rankling of church officials and, perhaps especially, the public confession of sin. They set out to rid the Anglican Church of corruption and incite a revival of holiness and spirituality. They were notoriously unruly and purposefully engaged in inappropriate behavior: the open defiance of church and local leaders and the disavowal of norms of comportment and mannered behavior that were central to southern Ugandan political and social life. Unlike neotraditionalists, revivalists' attitude toward moral reform was decidedly "cosmopolitan," invested in forging a new, worldly African Christian identity opposed to nativist movements like the Bataka Union. Derek Peterson, in his insightful history of the revival, has written that the revivalists "posed a threat to eastern Africa's patriotic organizers because they would not organize their lives around the spatial coordinates of their fatherlands."[31] This was a movement at odds with the patriotic traditionalists of the colonial era who sought to reassert the sexual and gendered norms of custom as the stabilizing force that would shepherd Africans into independence. But the revivalists were no less concerned with the politics of sex and family in colonial Uganda.

Like missionaries and traditionalist reformers, the revivalists sought to address the problems associated with an urban life where unrelated young women and men lived in close proximity and where formal marriage—either customary or Christian—had become harder to achieve and was more often delayed in favor of less formal domestic arrangements. The answer revivalists had was to embrace the practice of confession as a means of both personal and public reform. Public confessions drew large crowds who were compelled to watch the spectacle of individuals enumerating all sorts of inappropriate behavior and personal indiscretion. Women spoke publicly of their many lovers, men of their drunken trysts. This was not a practice common to either the subdued High Anglican cathedrals of downtown Kampala or to the Catholic Church, where confession was made discretely and only to a priest. Nor was it considered appropriate in precolonial Buganda, where such public, emotive displays of private life would have been considered disgraceful.[32] Public confession was a spectacle, one that thumbed its nose at the standards for decency, privacy, and deference that ruled public interaction in Ganda society. These were the problems of modern society laid bare, for all the world to see.

The revival provided an alternative narrative about how to address the problems of urbanization and the modern state. Rather than reassert the individual's place within traditional structures of clan and family, revivalists embraced a new form of self-fashioning. Public confession asserted the individual self, with all its capacity for sin and redemption, at the center of a project to craft a new type of moral ballast with which to navigate the modern world. This practice also sought to reimagine the place of the church within the colonial state. Since first setting foot in Buganda the Anglican Church had been a tool of the elite, a mechanism through which forms of precolonial power and privilege had been modified but also reasserted. The revival was an antielitist movement that sought to empower marginalized groups of women and youth and to create a narrative about their own power and influence that was based not in neotraditionalist models for moral behavior but in new modes of self-critique. Christian narratives of sin and salvation, good and evil, provided a new language with which to describe social problems and colonial politics. Revivalists' confessions also provided the means for youth to cast doubt on the new forms of power associated with elite men and provided women with a language with which to criticize the moral misdeeds and social transgressions of powerful elders.[33]

By the independence period the revival had ended, but its influence was felt for a long time in the Anglican Church, especially as young revivalists eventually matured into church leaders. By the turn of the twenty-first century the East African Revival was remembered as an antiestablishment movement in Uganda, one that had thumbed its nose at the power and privilege associated with both traditional leaders and elite Christians. It was, however, also still remembered for the "weird" behavior of its members—to use the words of one pastor I interviewed. The practice of public confession—the overt focus on public and personal reformation as the new basis for moral security and social reform—was never accepted by the larger public as "normal" behavior. Nevertheless, elements of the revival can be traced to present-day Christian activism and religious practice, though—as I will discuss below—new Christian movements have also sought to distance themselves from this controversial history.

The result of this series of debates spanning the central decades of colonial rule was that the family, and perhaps especially the sexual conduct at the center of marriage and domestic life, emerged as a point not only for concern but for political manipulation. Precolonial Ganda authority had been animated by the good management of personal relationships—between patron and client, leader and subject, and father and child. Power was perceived in an overt, everyday way as a moral project; it was cultivated and maintained in ways understood to be intimate, even emotionally resonant. As historian Carol Summers has argued, the kabaka's power was described in ways that emphasized his closeness to his subjects; he was "the husband to his chiefs as well as his wives."[34] In the colonial period concerns about the breakdown of these bonds—in particular through the commodification of land—were communicated in terms of arguments about the family and sexuality. The family became the locus of moral outrage over changing norms of power and status, and attempting to "reform" the family became a practice of serious political importance. Debating family life and the costs of sexual indiscretions was a way to make arguments about how power should be asserted and how the state was to be conceived. But these arguments took various, often contradictory, forms. One primary route was to reassert and reimagine a place for customs within the modern urban landscape. Another route, spearheaded by the revivalists, was to reject these nativist critiques and instead forge a new sort of moral politics, one focused on the reform of the self.

Politics always happens on "moral" terms, in arguments that challenge and attempt to assert ideas about public behavior and one's obligations to others. This may be one reason why arguments over sexuality and gender seem to appear so often at the center of political discourse in Africa—and elsewhere—today. During the postapartheid period, numerous scholars pointed to the ways in which sexuality and family life seemed to become the locus for struggles that sought to address the dramatic alteration to the social contract and the emerging pressures caused by new forms of economic exploitation in the new South African state.[35] Uganda's AIDS epidemic has helped outline another such moment, one in which political and social concerns have come into focus through arguments regarding the family and home. These are debates that draw from the longer history I have outlined here in which disparate groups have periodically attempted to forge new claims to a moral authority that would better both the family and society.

The Present-Day Politics of Moral Reform: Cultivating a Cosmopolitan Moral Authority

In Uganda, debates about the costs of modern attitudes about family life resurface daily. In 2013 the Parliament of Uganda debated the Marriage and Divorce Bill, a piece of legislation that sought certain legal protections for women in marriage. The bill mandated the division of property at the time of divorce, outlawed marital rape, and gave cohabiting partners shared property rights. It was heavily supported by the women's movement in Uganda because of the protections these new rights would extend to women, who under the current laws had little recourse to claim any part of shared marital property after a divorce. (In Uganda it is common for couples to keep property or assets registered only to one or the other spouse rather than register it jointly.) But the bill was fiercely opposed by Christians, with many pastors writing newspaper editorials and speaking out about the moral costs of making divorce "mandatory and automatic."[36] One born-again Christian I knew posted his displeasure with the bill on Facebook, suggesting it should be re-named the "Marriage *to* Divorce" bill. Establishing shared rights to property was mocked as an incitement to couples, and especially to women, to abandon marital unions. What was the good of a marriage if you could "gain" from a divorce? they asked. As an editorial in a national newspaper noted, "By em-phasising the division of family property between the couple at the time of divorce, the bill seems to undermine the importance of stable marriages and families in nation building. It sends a wrong message to wives that the short-cut to get rich quick is divorce."[37]

At the heart of these debates were questions about what sorts of mar-riages provide for more stable and more moral unions. While many in the women's movement saw the new bill as strengthening marriages, making them more equitable and just, many more Ugandans—especially religious leaders—saw the bill as a full-scale assault on marriage itself. The bill's de-tractors derided the idea of a marriage based on certain state-sanctioned rights and responsibilities; to them such a model seemed weak and open to easy dissolution. Concerns about the Marriage and Divorce Bill reveal a wider distrust of certain ways of thinking about individuals as social and moral beings. Echoing colonial-era debates over the protection of bridewealth, such concerns reveal how the bill's detractors felt that marriages founded on personal rights and individual desires seemed morally suspect and socially inappropriate. As in the 1920s "rehabilitation" of customary marriage, a strong union was considered to be one that was oriented toward more than the state alone; it was validated by cultural and religious practices that were believed to strengthen the marriage by making it more deeply rooted in social rela-tionships and more accountable to the broader community.

The Christian activist movement surrounding AIDS echoed many of these same tensions. It was a movement that gained strength from its promotion of a discourse that celebrated certain cultural traditions and values, especially as these were understood to strengthen Christian marriages and families. Be-ginning in the early years of the twenty-first century, born-again Christian churches in Kampala were increasingly active in social protests and educa-tion campaigns promoting abstinence and marital faithfulness as the primary defenses against the devastating epidemic. During the years of my fieldwork (2004–11), these churches often publicized the spectacular mass weddings of dozens of couples, all wearing white gowns and neat black suits. Such spectacles helped churches promote marriage as desirable, glamorous, and—in an era when many Ugandans delayed marriage because of the costs

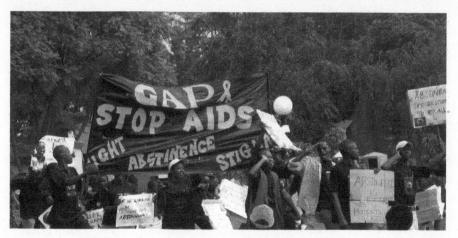

FIGURE 2.1. "Fight abstinence stigma"; Christian abstinence activists

associated with bridewealth and formal wedding receptions—accessible to all. Church leaders advocated marriage as a solution to society's problems: a panacea for broken homes, wayward youth, and unstable domestic unions. Marriage and family life became a core topic for sermons and workshops. Often these became public campaigns: youth rallies encouraging college students to "plan for marriage" and "fight abstinence stigma" were commonplace in Kampala during these years (see figure 2.1).

When I first lived in Kampala in the late 1990s, born-again Christians were not yet considered a powerful religious group, and many people distrusted the loud, charismatic church services that differed so greatly from the staid, formal services of the mainline churches.[38] The Anglican Church in particular was then considered (and remains) a path to status and power, and many older people wondered about young peoples' decision to abandon that path. But, as has happened over much of sub-Saharan Africa in recent decades, these churches have become not only increasingly popular but also politically influential; social activism within these churches has also become more common. Young people now participate in "campaigns" to promote social values and sexual morality. Increasingly these campaigns have aligned with legislative agendas, and the Ugandan parliament has recently seen the introduction of several controversial bills that seek to regulate sexuality and domestic life.[39] Born-again churches have effectively engaged a language of "tradition" to assert their own moral authority within the political sphere. Much more than a simple parroting of Western efforts, the political projects of Ugandan Christians have been successful because of the deft way these campaigns have infused Western ideals such as personal accountability into the language of tradition.

To argue that born-again churches celebrate a certain concept of traditional culture will seem at odds with most descriptions of African charismatic Christianity. Throughout the continent, Pentecostal and born-again churches are known for their rejection of traditionalist spirituality. Traditional practices, including certain family rituals, are often described as satanic and considered spiritually dangerous. Certain types of born-again prayer, described as "spiritual warfare," focus on the expulsion of "traditional" spirits from believers' bodies and souls. Tradition in many ways exists within a strict dichotomy, viewed in opposition to the modern Christian world. Often this is a dichotomy mapped spatially onto the rural-urban divide of contemporary African life. Traditional culture is viewed as backward, a hindrance to modern development. This is in many ways a view shared by non-Christian Ugandans. When I was last in Uganda, one of the most popular TV shows was a late-night Luganda language program that sought out stories about witchcraft, sorcery, and the traditional rituals still practiced in most of the country. The program took a lurid, sensationalist tone in their coverage of these practices. Tradition in this approach was made to be somewhat scandalous; it was associated with the unmodern, the poor, and the rural. In rejecting this idea and image of tradition, born-again churches forge a distinctly nonlocal, cosmopolitan identity. In Uganda this is an identity explicitly at odds with mainline churches (the Catholic and Anglican) whose authority structures draw from and refigure precolonial ones and whose orientations are distinctly local and national. Born-again churches eschew ethnic and national distinctions in an effort to forge a transnational Christian communion. In Uganda the symbolic representations of this identity are everywhere, from traveling American and German evangelists, to the row of international flags outside one Kampala megachurch, to another church's globe logo. Born-again Christianity's antitraditionalist stance effects a sense of spatial dislocation, reorienting believers within a global realm.

Yet a language of tradition and culture remain central to Christian political projects. Christian churches seek to become arbiters of personal morality and family life, defenders of specifically African or Ugandan values. The protests and political advocacy engaged in by the Christian communities I knew in Kampala sought to define and defend a selective idea of "traditional culture," of female submission, wifely virtue, and monogamy that, like the practices of the moral reformers that preceded them, viewed the family as a point of political intervention that gained its authority from its unstable claim to a reified "cultural" past. More than a reiteration of American politics, such arguments drew on a particularly Ugandan history in which such claims to authentic tradition provided the means for moral social reform.

Ruth Marshall has called Pentecostalism a "prescriptive regime" that works on and through the self to address shifting forms of authority in contemporary Africa.[40] It does so by placing special focus on maintaining the state of salvation and warding off the ever-present power of Satan and ungodly forces. Being born again demands constant attention to the spiritual struggles that give shape to one's lived experience; by participating in prayer, healing services, and practices of deliverance and prophecy, believers may address and withstand physical and material affliction. These are "techniques of the self" in the Foucauldian sense, and they are practices that give shape to a born-again moral subjectivity. In this sense, a born-again politics seems at first to be one intensely focused on the moral fashioning of the individual. But the pursuit of religious virtues also demands that Christians seek to inspire others to accept salvation. Born-again Christians in Kampala view themselves as more socially active than their mainline Christian counterparts; they organize university student forays into city slums; they "adopt" children from the camps of internally displaced people in northern Uganda and neighboring children with HIV. They view the process of individual self-fashioning to be a socially "ambitious" project,[41] one that seeks to engage others through the personal pursuit of such Christian virtues as compassion, grace, and love.

The private nature of born-again politics works to separate their ambitions from the derided, supposedly immoral realm of everyday state politics. The social outreach of these churches focuses on the antithesis to the political; theirs is a politics of the home and family, driven by Christian love rather than worldly ambition. The authority that the churches claim in their efforts to address social problems is an authority that draws from the power that kinship and family still hold in the lives of nearly all Ugandans. Born-again churches promise youth the ability to learn how to better "manage" and remake the family. It is a position that acknowledges traditional forms of authority—perhaps especially patriarchy—but also seeks to make this traditional institution into a "modern" one. Certain aspects of traditional life may be discarded or refashioned while others are celebrated.

In their embrace of what might be termed a "conservative cosmopolitan" identity, born-again Ugandan youth undermine analyses that view Pentecostal/charismatic Christianity as a homogenizing influence in Africa or that sets the Christian identity against a traditional Ugandan identity.[42] Struggles over youth identity fit within a larger narrative of Christianity in which negotiations between Ugandan and Western ways of behaving as "proper" persons have already played out. The debates raised today concerning family roles, hierarchies of age and gender, and sexual morality have their precedents in the Ugandan "moral crises" of the colonial era that I have recounted earlier in this chapter; in that era, changing standards of obligation and reciprocity created a sense of social upheaval strikingly similar to that of modern times. These periods of moral debate and struggle have resulted not in the emergence of clearly opposed categories of Christian persons and traditional Ganda ones; instead they have played an integral role in the reshaping and overlap of both categories.

The social projects of born-again AIDS activists draw upon powerful and deeply significant arguments about the nature of authentic forms of authority within social and political realms. In their efforts to "work on" traditional institutions and emphasize the power of family relationships, churches began to more forcefully engage the political realm in the late twentieth and early twenty-first centuries. In certain ways contemporary born-again Christianity reflects the intense emphasis on social reform and personal responsibility seen in the midcentury revivalists who rejected "tradition." And yet, perhaps surprisingly, born-again Christians also demonstrate a keen appreciation of the moral virtues of a claim to traditional legitimacy and authority, a claim to tradition that has not been forged through traditional spiritual ties (which have been vehemently rejected) or tied to a sense of ethnic solidarity. It is an authority drawn from a revival of family and kin relationships as the authentic source of a moral and social equilibrium that can ensure prosperity. In their public emphasis on sexual morality and family life, born-again Christians seek to develop a political stance based in older forms of moral legitimacy, even as they seek to transform the shape traditional institutions take.

Conclusion: Clans, Kinship, and the Politics of Ugandan Families

Jane Guyer and Samuel Belinga have studied the focus on kinship in the African ethnographic record to argue that the intense interest in the political economy of lineage in studies of precolonial Africa has overstated its importance, and obscured other forms of precolonial political mobilization. If kinship has been constructed as a focus of ethnographers and historians, it is in part, Guyer and Belinga argue, because it was an institution in place during the colonial era, when the European study of African societies began to intensify.[43] The historical scholarly significance of kinship was ensured in part due to its endurance in spite of the force of the colonial state. Yet for Africans themselves the importance of the clan and kin group is not merely a scholarly construction. For those living under colonial rule, the family became a critical idea to "think with" and with which to contest new forms of state power. With explicit colonial control over other forms of precolonial political authority (in Buganda, most especially kingship) the kin group became more important as a political force. Furthermore, the changes to political power experienced during the colonial era were morally destabilizing. As the brief history I have traced herein reveals, Ugandans' reactions to their changing relationships to the state were often couched in terms of concerns about their family lives. The family was viewed as a morally stabilizing force in the face of social disruption; kinship and lineage groups provided a sense of social continuity during a period of political crisis. The combination of these factors resulted in the kin group (and, perhaps also in Buganda, the clan[44]) emerging as an ever more important repository of an older type of political authority that drew its power from the moral obligations between leaders and followers. Even as the family has been dramatically transformed throughout the twentieth century, it remains a concept that carries deep significance and retains the ability to mobilize people around notions of the morality of power and the necessity of certain "traditional" institutions as ballast for the modern state.

Born-again Christians have claimed their own version of kin-based moral authority as they seek to reform society through a focus on youth sexuality, family life, and marriage. On the one hand, born-again Christians engage "traditional" life from a distance; theirs is an effort to preserve but also reform Ugandan ideas about the family and marriage and to make them modern. In doing so, their efforts connect them to an emergent and powerful form of global Christian politics that seems to now extend its reach from Houston to Kampala to Lagos and beyond. On the other hand, as much as they have adopted a cosmopolitan worldview, Ugandan born-again Christians consider projects of moral reform through a decidedly local lens. For such Christians, the moral authority to forge new models of family life come from the protection of certain ideas about the significance of the interrelationships among social actors, the traditional value of interdependence, and the moral obligations vested in relationships of kin and clientage. The Ugandan Christian effort to promote abstinence and "faithfulness" is thus animated by something more than the American ideal of accountability, especially as such accountability is interpreted by Americans to mean self-sufficiency and autonomy in decisions about health and wellness. This is a tension that animated Ugandan Christian AIDS protests and came to shape why and how the American messages of abstinence and faithfulness were interpreted and put into use by Ugandans. In the following chapters I will explore how such conflicts were navigated by youth seeking ways to be moral, modern persons in the midst of the AIDS epidemic.

THE CONTEXT OF A POLICY

PART II

❖

Engagements

3 "ABSTINENCE IS FOR ME, HOW ABOUT YOU?"
The Meaning and Morality of Sex

One of the most provocative moments in the debates about AIDS prevention in Uganda might have been Kabaka Mutebi's promise in 2004 that all young Baganda women who abstained from sex until they were married would receive a washing machine as a wedding gift from the Buganda kingdom.[1] There is much one could analyze in Mutebi's promise, but most striking may be the symbolic effort to link a girl's virginity to the ultimate material icon of domestic virtue. To remain a virgin, by this calculation, was not only about protecting oneself from HIV—or even cultivating one's "traditional values"; it was also about pursuing a path of upward mobility, a path that promised a more modern, "developed," and secure future. In many Ugandan communities the choice to abstain was a choice that was often reframed in terms of a similar calculus, one that weighed personal aspirations against present-day desires. On one billboard displayed near Makerere University in 2007, and funded by the U.S. President's Emergency Plan for AIDS Relief (PEPFAR), the question ABSTINENCE IS FOR ME, HOW ABOUT YOU? was accompanied by photos of young adults in graduation gowns or carrying stacks of books (see figure 3.1). The message was clear enough: abstaining is a method of achieving one's goals, a surer path to coveted university degrees and steady employment. This was a message at the heart of PEPFAR's focus on "behavior change," a message rooted in an ethos of self-improvement through self-control.

This section of the book, part 2, concerns the ways young people have heard but transformed the American message that becoming more "accountable" for one's decisions regarding sex would make a person healthier and less likely to become infected with HIV. I argued in chapter 1 that personal accountability became a dominant principle that guided American approaches to humanitarian and development aid at the beginning of the twenty-first

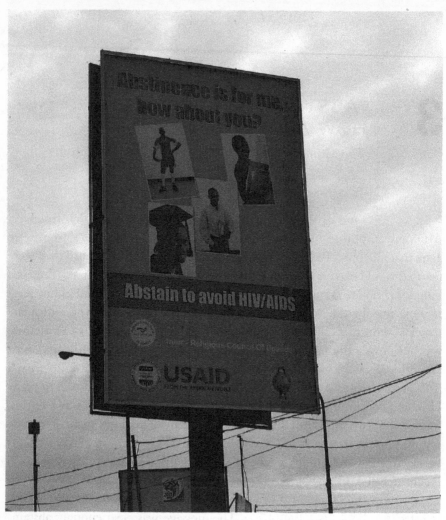

FIGURE 3.1. "Abstinence is for me, how about you?"

century. This was an approach that was animated by particular values and ideals—especially the moral worth of personal empowerment and autonomy—that were considered socially transformative. Accountability from the American perspective was understood to be a way of ordering and managing approaches to international aid and justifying donor programs by imagining the transformative effects of American "compassion." For Ugandans, however, the message of accountability was engaged relative to a broader array of concerns surrounding contemporary and historical experiences of sexuality, family life, and gender relations. In this and the next two chapters I examine how this message about personal accountability was taken up and transformed by Ugandan activists. What did it mean to "abstain and be faithful," and why was this message appealing to youth in Uganda? What did personal accountability come to stand for in relation to other ways of acting ethically in contemporary Uganda?

Moral values underlie the message of abstinence and faithfulness, but these values were not inevitably and consistently reproduced as the policy circulated from the United States to Uganda. In Uganda the ethical conflict that defined the choice to abstain was not, as it might have been in the United States, framed only as a choice between good and bad behaviors—that is, an attempt to avoid, in the Christian sense, a sinful mistake driven by the weakness of human desire. Rather, abstinence was experienced as a struggle to define moral personhood itself. What sorts of relationships are deemed productive and proper? How is moral behavior identified and pursued? As I noted in chapter 2, these debates were formed against a backdrop where "traditional values" were topics of continual debate and reflection among ordinary Ugandans. Family life, marriage, and sexual norms were understood to be in a state of change, and a variety of social actors were invested in forwarding and defending interpretations of what parts of traditional culture and modern life were worth redeeming.

In this chapter, I analyze abstinence as an ethical practice that provided youth the means to navigate between two competing models of moral personhood that coexisted in Uganda: a neoliberal message about sexual autonomy and personal accountability, and an older model of sexual respectability that highlighted young people's interdependence and obligations to kin group and clan. Abstinence was understood to be a pathway to certain measures of modern success, but young people's opinions about abstinence also revealed a deep ambivalence toward aspects of modern relationships—especially values that emphasized personal freedom and desire. Young people criticized modern relationships driven by uncontrolled lust and personal interest as dangerous and destabilizing. At the same time, youth were also critical of "traditional" models for sexual behavior—those they characterized as driven more by obligation than love." Abstinence was a "technique of the self" that allowed youth to navigate, critique, and bridge competing models for ethical behavior and moral personhood that coexisted in Uganda.

My analysis in this chapter focuses on the Ugandan Christian concept of "intentional" relationships and the ways this ideal form of intimacy has colored youth perceptions of abstinence. Abstinence, especially in American frameworks, has been frequently presented as a choice that could withdraw youth from all sexually intimate relationships. It has been a message about "investing" in oneself to become, as the billboard depicted, better educated and more successful. But in the years I lived in Kampala and conducted field-work there, I found that abstinence's appeal actually lay in how it provided young adults with a discourse about relationships that emphasized youth agency and choice: it became a way for them to think about how to manage, rather than withdraw completely, from sexual and intimate bonds. This colored the ways youth thought about the nature of sexual intimacy with peers and how they viewed relationships with their parents and other family members. As opposed to a straightforward moral discourse about sexual "self-control," abstinence was appealing because it provided young people with the means to consider the shape of their intimate lives. The ways they talked about abstinence reflected a complex moral terrain on which they weighed competing models for sexual morality. The ways youth discussed abstinence, and embraced the practice, challenged assumptions about the predictable replication of American messages about sexual risk that would follow from PEPFAR's influence.

Many criticisms of abstinence as an HIV prevention strategy have pointed out the ways that the decision to abstain may be limited by what are called structural factors such as economic inequality, gender and family relations, and physical insecurity (for instance, the prevalence of domestic violence).[2] That is, even if a person wants to abstain, other factors may limit his or her ability to do so. This chapter acknowledges and moves beyond such criticisms to examine what abstinence meant within the Ugandan context at the start of this century: Why and for whom was it appealing and possible to abstain? What did this practice mean and represent in the Ugandan context? Decisions about sex are, of course, limited by financial and social considerations, but they are also shaped by moral evaluations and attitudes about what sex is and does. In the following pages I explore how abstinence fit into and helped shift the experience of youth sexuality in Kampala, generating new conflicts surrounding sex and exposing the limits of abstinence as an AIDS prevention strategy within a community that had embraced it. I begin with a description of one of the communities at the center of the abstinence movement in Kampala: University Hill Church.

By 2006, when I began spending time there, University Hill Church (UHC) was devoted to the promotion of youth abstinence.[3] Its congregation was small compared to other urban born-again Christian churches in Uganda, with only a few hundred regular members and a core group of perhaps several dozen young adults who attended weekly prayer meetings and church programs. Sunday services usually drew about two or three hundred people. Most of the congregation was drawn from the university, where many students learned about the church from UHC's on-campus programs and outreach activities. During the period of my fieldwork the church maintained offices near the campus, in a pair of neighboring rented houses, one of which was nicknamed the White House, a title brandished in black paint across the white building's facade. Behind this building there was an open-air prayer shelter with wooden floors and a metal roof that the congregation had christened the Pentagon, so named because it was here that church members conducted spiritual warfare by harnessing the force of collective prayer to address spiritual and social problems. Youth who regularly attended the church would gather in these buildings, studying and chatting before class, often congregating around the worn reception desk inside the front door of the White House. Midday prayer and weekly Bible study were held in the Pentagon, which was the largest meeting area outside the rented space used for Sunday services. Several of the most dedicated students were hired as interns and spent most of their free time at the White House, managing the front desk and running errands for UHC's leadership. The manager of the church—the pastor's "right-hand man"—was Robert, a man in his mid-twenties who, rumor had it, had declined a job offer at a large international nongovernmental organization (NGO) to work for the church's pastor—a decision that signaled both his devotion to the pastor and his commitment to the church as a path of upward mobility. One of his duties was to hire and manage the student interns, who were paid small sums of money for their service (when it was available, about twenty dollars per month or so, with extra for lunch and transport costs). The interns were the most active members of the church, and I came to know many of them well.

As in other parts of Africa, born-again Christians in Uganda form an increasingly influential constituency both in Kampala and throughout the countryside. Churches like UHC are part of a larger wave of charismatic and Pentecostal Christianity that has been growing in the Global South since at least the mid-1990s.[4] Most of these newer Christian churches are set against the mainline, colonial-era churches that preceded them and are distinguished from earlier charismatic movements by their expressly "global" outlook.[5] For youth, participation in a globally oriented church defined less by relationships to colonial or state institutions and more by relationships with Christian communities and economies abroad was powerfully appealing. Membership in an urban born-again church indicated belonging to a *particular* cosmopolitan community that was largely predicated on its critical stance toward both an older generation's traditionalism (and its mainline Christianity) and secular modern culture.

UHC was founded by a charismatic Ganda pastor, Thomas Walusimbi, who told me he had started the church to address the issue of youth "sexual purity." He had begun his career in the early 1990s, at the height of the AIDS epidemic, as a youth pastor. He himself, like many other Ugandans, had suffered personal losses due to the epidemic, and felt called to dedicate his ministry to the issues surrounding AIDS. In 1998 he founded his own church, and the following year he moved it to the Wandegeya neighborhood in Kampala, one that is frequented by the young adults and university students he wished to attract to his congregation. While Walusimbi's focus on AIDS prevention preceded the advent of PEPFAR, his and his church's prominence and purpose expanded in the years after the U.S. government and American Christians mobilized in support of AIDS prevention. In the early years of the new century Walusimbi cultivated his image as a local expert in Christian AIDS education. By 2003, when PEPFAR was being developed, he was already known to members of the administration of President George W. Bush as a Ugandan involved in abstinence promotion. He told me he had served as a kind of expert consultant on Ugandan sexuality and AIDS prevention programs for several Americans who testified before Congress in support of PEPFAR. He also traveled to Washington, DC, to participate in such events as the National Prayer Breakfast, an annual meeting that serves as a networking opportunity not only for American politicians but also for the numerous foreign Christian leaders who attend as invited guests.[6] In the wake of PEPFAR's launch Walusimbi's church founded an NGO that received a small grant through the program to support abstinence and faithfulness education. The NGO's primary PEPFAR-funded project was to produce a newspaper-style publication about abstinence that was distributed on the university campus.[7]

Despite these seemingly high-powered connections, Walusimbi had a much smaller church infrastructure and congregation than did most high-profile Ugandan pastors. UHC was run on a modest budget, with no permanent church buildings; all office and worship spaces were rented. To support the congregation Walusimbi relied in part on his relationships with American church congregations and individual American Christian donors whose interest in UHC grew as African AIDS prevention became a higher-profile Christian cause in the United States. Financial gifts from abroad were quite modest, on the order of several thousand dollars annually, but they far exceeded the amount of money the church was able to collect from its own congregation in the form of tithes and pledges.[8] In addition to direct gifts, American church groups would also sponsor specific programs, such as the Christian leadership symposium on Makerere's campus that I attended in 2007 or the youth mission to teach abstinence in rural schools I observed that same year. UHC would benefit from such programs by helping facilitate or host the visiting Americans. Abstinence was an important focus of the church because church leaders viewed it as their Christian mission and also because it was a cause that raised the church's local and international profiles, drawing in critical forms of financial aid.[9]

If abstinence was the focus of many of the church's programs, UHC was also defined by its close connection to the state university, where many of UHC's members attended school. The young people at UHC represented a more diverse range of backgrounds than might have been found among a group of Makerere University students even a decade earlier. In 2006–7, during the primary years of my fieldwork, Makerere University was struggling through a period of intense change, one that had been defined by the attempt of university administrators to adopt a market-oriented approach to education that reduced the number of government scholarships available in favor of recruiting tuition-paying students and emphasizing the "commercialization" of courses of study, especially in the Faculty of Arts.[10] The introduction of private tuition-paying students had dramatically expanded the student population at Makerere, increasing it fivefold between 1992 and 2003 and opening higher education to a wider range of Ugandan students than ever before. The massive influx of students had strained campus resources, and most students lived off-campus in student hostels or low-cost rented rooms rather than in the campus dormitories. Lecture halls were regularly overflowing, and campus facilities struggled to accommodate the rapidly expanding student population. Perhaps most significantly, these reforms had greatly reduced the percentage of students receiving government aid, placing the burden of the cost of education on students and their families.

Most students I knew lived in perpetually precarious financial situations, scrambling from term to term to find the resources necessary to pay tuition, fees, and general costs of living. Few of the students who attended UHC had attended the preparatory schools that had for decades been the preferred feeder schools for Makerere and had long served the children of Uganda's elite and powerful. Many students now came from rural families who had scrambled to pay the tuition at one of the many new for-profit secondary schools opening throughout the nation; others had graduated from less prestigious upcountry boarding schools. In many ways, higher education was far more accessible than it had been in the past. Yet for all of the professionalization of the university experience students still faced high rates of unemployment upon graduation and, much like in many Western countries today, young people cycled in and out of school as their financial circumstances allowed them to in an effort to attain some better combination of diplomas or degrees or to put off the inevitability of unemployment. On campus, the catchphrases "entrepreneurial spirit" and "leadership development" proliferated uneasily alongside the reality of unemployment and the sense that degrees with new names held no guarantee of financial success. The university remained—as it had long been—a site of idealized striving, but the effects of new financial and academic policies had contributed to a sense that, like other new forms of wealth and success in Kampala, the distinction granted by one's degree had an intangible, chimera-like quality.

Born-again Christian churches like UHC sought to address young people's sense of frustration directly by emphasizing a discourse of personal empowerment and self-help through God. Distinct from the "prosperity gospel" popular throughout Africa and North America, which emphasizes a spiritual, "magical" relationship between faith and material wealth,[11] the gospel of self-help that proliferated in Kampala's English-speaking churches during my years of research emphasized the cultivation of embodied dispositions that were believed to generate success: personal vision, planning, and an intense understanding of individual skill sets and goals. This was in many ways a spiritual lesson infused with the language of neoliberal reform, one in which greater faith would lead to more self-control and eventually personal empowerment and success. Support for abstinence fit into this ethos easily; its promotion in many ways echoed the rubric of "developing faith" that Daromir Rudnyckyj uses to describe Islamic corporate development programs in Indonesia.[12] In born-again churches, as in Rudnyckyj's training seminars, faith was viewed as a mechanism that helped cultivate new ethical dispositions that would enable economic development and success during a period of perceived moral crisis. But the optimistic images of entrepreneurial self-empowerment that seemed to be proliferating in Kampala and on university campuses were shadowed by the sense that these messages espoused a path to prosperity that lay out of reach for most. More troublingly, the emphasis on self-reliance familiar to schoolgoing youth existed uneasily alongside alternative rubrics for success that emphasized obligations to family and clan and the management of hierarchical patronage ties. Abstinence emphasized a "working on the self" that reshaped young people's relationships with those around them, and in this way it was received as a radical message. It was a discourse about behavior that echoed, but also clearly diverged from, older techniques of the self that had long defined moral conduct in Buganda and Uganda. This was central to abstinence's appeal, but this distinction also outlined the limits of the strategy's reach and exacerbated the conflicts inherent in its embrace.

Disciplined Selves: Two Perspectives on Sex and Moral Behavior

During a weeklong seminar for secondary school students held in the cavernous auditorium of a recently built private high school in Mukono, a suburb of Kampala, the image of a "fortress" emerged as a frequent theme in lessons about abstinence. I had traveled to the conference after meeting one of its American organizers at a World AIDS Day rally in Kampala. Michael was a white American in his early thirties who worked as a missionary in eastern Africa and traveled extensively to lead workshops on abstinence for African youth. He was excited by his work, revved up in the presence of African Christians who were also so clearly dedicated to the cause of abstinence as AIDS prevention. He encouraged me to join him in Mukono, where he was meeting up with other foreign missionaries to run a workshop for high school students.

During one of the more memorable sessions that day, several of the workshop leaders constructed the outline of a "fortress" on the floor (see figure 3.2). The cardboard circle, large enough to fit two people standing inside it—was covered with slogans and words that were meant to represent "marriage." Marriage was a "security fence, fortress, boundary, legal limit, protection" that surrounded a married couple, making sex "safe." I was familiar with such language, as the youth at UHC were similarly taught ways to protect themselves through prayer by imagining their bodies covered in an "armor of God," a barrier that would help them control their desires and abstain.

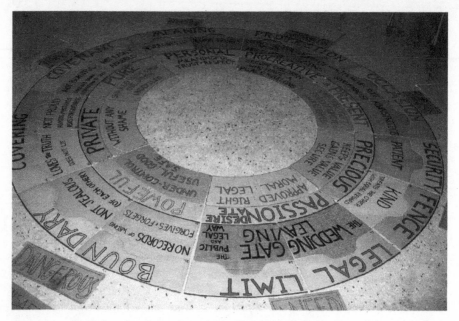

FIGURE 3.2. "Marriage is a fortress"; Mukono abstinence workshop, January 2007

Similarly, in church skits a "wall" was often used to describe marriage, sometimes visually represented by a ring of church members surrounding a fictional married couple. Pastors would remind youth that intimate relationships should be "in your control" and unwanted relationships and demands on the person should be "cast off." These images, which emphasized abstinence as a pathway to a marriage that would cut off the couple from the demands of others, seemed radical in a society where the maintenance and cultivation of relationships of interdependence define moral behavior and moral personhood. As I discussed in chapter 2, marriage—perhaps more than any other relationship in Uganda—was articulated by the network of family, kin, and clan relationships that gave that union shape. To characterize it as a bond that separated the couple from others—as this image of the "fortress" did—was surprising given what I knew about Ugandan marriages.

Abstinence was often described by Ugandans—especially older officials and pastors—as a return to "traditional" sexual norms. But such claims were complicated by images like those presented in this workshop. These lessons about the benefits of sexual "self-control" highlighted the ways that abstinence was a strategy animated by particular moral values—autonomy, independence, and personal choice. The meanings attributed to this model of the disciplined sexual subject diverged from older ideals as often as they reinforced them, and these were ways of thinking about sex and sexual relationships that were not universally shared by Ugandans. As I sat in that auditorium, surrounded by restless high school students, I began to think about how these lessons on marital fidelity and sexual "self-control" made sense (or didn't) within Ugandan frameworks for sexual behavior. I realized that many of the images these well-meaning missionaries were using were ones developed for an American audience; they were animated by certain attitudes about sex that had a particular cultural history not wholly familiar to this Ugandan audience.

In Faramerz Dabhoiwala's history of Western sexuality, he notes that the contemporary Euro-American orientation toward sex, where it is considered a matter of private, personal concern governed by Christian ideas about personal conscience and sin, is an early modern manifestation that dates to the Reformation.[13] With the cultivation of an idea of religious freedom in the early eighteenth century there also emerged the sense that individual conscience should govern moral conduct. Dabhoiwala writes, "This gradual elevation of personal instinct as the supreme moral arbiter was one of the most striking conceptual developments of the period."[14] This was, he notes, a remarkable change in how moral conduct was both imagined and measured; it was a shift that oriented the experience of personhood inward, demarcating the outlines of the modern individual. Enlightenment-era philosophical thought, perhaps especially the Kantian emphasis on rational choice as the foundation for ethical life, further elaborated the idea that individual autonomy defined the moral being. The ways we have come to think about the individual as a locus for social action, perhaps especially so in modern times, reflects this history. Such a focus on personal agency, interior transformation, and sincerity of belief also articulates a particularly individualized view of personhood that is still widely viewed as characteristic of Christianity.[15] This is the "moral narrative of modernity" that Webb Keane describes in his study of Indonesian Protestantism—the emergence of the modern perspective on individual agency as imbued with moral virtue.[16] Talal Asad and others have argued that this construction of moral agency has played a role in how we view everything from contemporary human rights advocacy to global approaches to developmental aid and economic restructuring.[17]

This is a discourse about moral development and personal agency that also, in part, underlies and gives shape to experiences of abstinence within churches like UHC. To practice sexual abstinence is a process that directs

"Abstinence Is for Me, How about You?"

reflection about moral conduct inward, motivated by a desire to resist sinful temptation. Sexual prohibitions in Uganda are certainly not new, but what was new about the Christian project of abstinence was that it sought to outline a form of the (Christian) person and distinguish that form from other ways of being a sexually ethical subject. The struggle to abstain was imagined as an internal battle, one that required the closing off or "fortifying" of the individual or married couple from the demands and temptations of an external world.

In Ugandan society the experience of moral personhood was not oriented inward; rather, it emphasized a person's interdependence to others, both physically and spiritually. The distinction between African models of personhood (which are seen to emphasize social relatedness and embeddedness) and individualistic Christian ones has long been debated by scholars.[18] Charles Piot, writing about Kabre personhood, articulates this contrast: "Persons here do not 'have' relations, they 'are' relations."[19] Piot means to highlight how, in many African societies, the experience of the self—of illness, emotion, even personality—is frequently understood in terms of one's external relations rather than as a distinctive, set-apart, autonomous interiority. In this sense ethical reflection is not primarily a function of the tension generated by the Christian concept of sinfulness—the internal struggle generated between the righteous and fallen elements of every human soul. Rather, ethical reflection is turned outward in a way that demands interrogation of one's relationships with and responsibilities to others. In Ugandan cultures, the ceremonies that mark life stages and outline the available categories of social persons gain their meaning from an emphasis on the person's place within and responsibilities to the larger social group and lineage. The recognition of and investment in hierarchical relationships of kinship and clientism have long defined the path to social status and influence in Ugandan society, and the appearance that one has abandoned or ignored such relational obligations still stokes intense moral criticism and rebuke.[20]

This is not to say that the relational self is never a part of Christian and Western experiences of personhood, or that Africans do not orient themselves toward some construction of the individual. Nor do I mean to argue that "traditional" personhood and sexual behavior are vested with some static, immutable authority in the lives of Ugandans; quite the contrary. What anthropologists have long sought to highlight through these distinctions are the ways dominant Western frameworks of social action—concepts that celebrate the moral worth of autonomy, for instance—must be historically and culturally contextualized.[21] Assumptions about the universality of such constructs may be particularly problematic for the ways in which they obscure our understanding of alternative ethical practices.[22] They may also cloud our understanding of how local communities make sense of and repurpose "global" projects predicated on a moral message about individual behavior that emphasizes autonomy and accountability—especially in the realms of sexuality and health.

In most of eastern Africa the demonstration of self-restraint, modesty, and proper decorum have long been essential aspects of adult behavior. But in these societies self-restraint has more often reflected a concern for the external maintenance of moral community rather than an internal struggle over one's soul. Initiation ceremonies throughout the region created adults who knew "how to behave";[23] they were responsible for maintaining relationships of respect and deference (especially through the demonstration of modesty or avoidance) among dependent social groups. In Buganda, the ethnic region of Uganda that includes Kampala, the actualization of moral personhood is perhaps best expressed in the ideal of *ekitiibwa*, which is most commonly translated in everyday speech as "respectability" or "respect." The historian John Iliffe has written extensively about the ways this Ganda ideal fits alongside other models for "honor" in African societies; in his chapter on ekitiibwa he notes that this concept emphasized the ambition at the core of public behavior and comportment in precolonial Buganda.[24] Ekitiibwa was, for men, a combination of both bravery and loyalty, a way of conducting oneself that reinforced relationships of clientism and hierarchy that were essential aspects of political and personal life in the kingdom. This ideal was and remains so central to Ganda notions of proper behavior that it is sometimes translated simply as "morality."[25] Today in Buganda and many surrounding regions,[26] the term *ekitiibwa* is often used to describe the proper behavior of a spouse—the obedience, modesty, and faithfulness of a wife or the devotion a good husband demonstrates through the material support of his wife and children.

The ideal of ekitiibwa reveals how in much of precolonial Uganda self-control was an embodied state that was directed outward and used to mark and strengthen relationships. The moral worth of self-control was in the ways it reinforced and helped demarcate relationships of social interdependence and hierarchy. Rules governing respect and avoidance imposed special restraints on the display of sexuality and intimacy in particular. For instance, in Buganda ethical sexual behavior was (and mostly still is) marked by prohibitions against certain types of intimate interactions, such as any display of

"Abstinence Is for Me, How about You?"

familiarity (touching, eye contact) between sons-in-law and mothers-in-law. Because such rules of avoidance were meant to actualize broader networks of moral obligation and dependence, breeches of sexual taboos were considered to be both spiritually and socially threatening not only to the individuals involved but also to the larger kin group.[27] Rules of avoidance highlighted how a "well-mannered" person used sexual self-control to invest in and help reproduce the relationships of interdependence and obligation that gave shape to social life. Throughout Uganda self-restraint in sexual matters, and the control of sex and reproduction through varying practices of marriage, initiation, and terminal abstinence on the part of seniors, was key to traditional notions of both moral personhood and social reproduction.[28]

Given this broader context it is clear that Ugandans might have viewed a lesson about abstinence through a variety of lenses. Certainly for elders, such as Kabaka Mutebi or Yoweri Museveni, there was an effort to draw parallels between the idea of "abstinence" being touted by international public health officials and the older Ugandan ideas about ekitiibwa and traditional moral behavior. Pastor Walusimbi of UHC drew these parallels himself when he discussed with me how abstinence emerged as part of Uganda's prevention agenda:

> Virginity is a major value. Sexual restraint is a major core value of all our cultures. Marriage to a virgin is supposed to be celebrated with a goat.[29] In the eighties there was a new group of politicians [Museveni's government] who were trying to rebuild the nation. They came in as Marxists with a sense of discipline that was built off of "I care for others," that idea of common good, and "I need to sacrifice." And it rhymed well with a Christian ethic. So when HIV/AIDS broke out it was very easy to say "self-restraint," "sexual restraint." We all, the president, all of us. So the message of abstinence is really a message of sexual restraint.

Pastor Walusimbi drew a number of connections here—from cultural values to African socialism to Christian ethics—that, he argued, all support a model of "sexual restraint."[30] But the connections he and many others made take much for granted. The previous pages have emphasized how Ganda cultural ideals of ethical sexual behavior may be actualized differently from Christian or, for that matter, socialist ones. In this sense, for born-again Christian youth abstinence may be appealing for all the ways is it viewed as *different* from lessons about traditional "respectability." Interpreting abstinence as a lesson about self-reliance and sexual autonomy—creating a "fortress" from the personal demands of kin and clan—distinguishes it as a pathway to sexual discipline that for youth may be distinctly more appealing than traditional paths. From this perspective, abstinence could be viewed as a way for youth to not merely reproduce their elders' ideas about ethical sexuality but to engage, and sometimes criticize, those ideas.

Discussions about abstinence also helped youth establish a critique of modern attitudes about sexuality and highlighted a set of concerns about the contemporary era's effects on gender and sex. Specifically, abstinence was often presented as a means for managing, or keeping at bay, the myriad temptations and demands of modern life while at the same time cultivating other seemingly modern sensibilities like independence and what members of UHC called intentionality. It was a practice that allowed young adults to contemplate and debate ideas about what it meant to be a modern, moral sexual subject. Rather than cast off arguments that framed abstinence as a traditional value, young people used abstinence to criticize and consider a variety of models for ideal sexuality.

The appeal of abstinence lay in the way it could be used to navigate and resolve conflicting messages about what types of sexual relationships and family lives were moral. In a culture in which youth received multiple messages about what constituted moral behavior, abstinence was embraced as a way for them to talk about the conflicts they faced regarding their own sexuality and the problems they associated with both modern and traditional values. I will return later to the ways abstinence engaged with the notion of Ugandan tradition, but in the section below I focus on the ways abstinence was animated by fears and desires associated with modern sexuality.

The Moral Costs of Modern Sex

The pursuit of abstinence was set against a way of behaving that many Ugandans criticized. There was a widespread perception (one not necessarily new) that young people in Uganda were being persuaded to pursue a different way of life, one oriented away from their elders' influence and toward a more depraved, less morally sound, "foreign" way of being. When I ate lunch with Pastor Walusimbi at a local restaurant he insisted that the proprietors turn off the television while he was present. He explained that the TV, which had been showing popular music videos, was an example of what was wrong in Ugandan society: "I am actually thinking that the chickens are coming home to roost. Look at East African TV. It's coming home to roost. Now we have kids who don't care about self-respect because they are raised on pornography, sexual addiction, sexuality. . . . I just think that the seeds of ungodliness that have been sowed from the West are coming forth in manifestations." Pastor Walusimbi expressed a popular sentiment about youth culture. Youth were disrespectful, even "out of control" because they were being swayed by a way of life that was not their own; they were ceding to an authority, represented by urban discos and sexuality-laden media, that was alien—and opposed—to their parents' authority.

Life in the city has long generated such fears in Uganda, as it has, of course, in other parts of the world. The city, and perhaps especially the university, was marked by the sense that it was a place where many traditional forms of social control and authority were absent or weak. Young people at UHC would tell me they feared that many of their peers were "lost" in a city that provided too many temptations. They would criticize the proliferation of addictions among their friends, the sense that young people had little control over their desires and that this loss of control was destabilizing. In an editorial in UHC's newspaper one male church member appealed for more pornography filters on the university's computer system to combat the proliferation of this sexual "addiction." After describing in detail what he felt was the extensive consumption of pornography on campus he ended his article with the plea, "Without any further intervention this generation is destined for disaster. We gently appeal to the Makerere University administration to Help [sic] with pornography filters."

The message of abstinence was inseparable from these fears. Its practitioners believed that it provided a way of acting and comporting oneself so as to ward off the dangers of the city—the loss of control, the absorption into addiction—that were the focus of so many warning testimonials in the village and the church. But these messages differed from the scolding cries of elders who blamed young people for HIV. In the eyes of the youth at UHC, abstinence was not experienced as a return to "traditional" behaviors and relationships; it was understood to be a rational, quite modern calculation through which time, energy, and money were conserved in pursuit of other life goals. The banner hanging over a group of actors during a church performance read DOUBLE YO' PLEASURE! MULTIPLY YO' HAPPINESS! Part of this message referred to the argument that if you waited to have sex—so the story went—the sex you did have would be much more pleasurable. But the banner also spoke to the idea that abstinence promised a new method of success through which investing in self-control in the present would reap greater returns in the future. Abstinence was understood to be a very modern behavior that would help young people manage modern vices.

In an article about dating in the church newspaper one young man expressed this sentiment: "Those who date carelessly lack focus though they say they do it for fun. Friends in that category tell me they date and go for those short term relationships because they want someone to eat their money." Dating—however "fun"—is not a winning proposition in this young man's opinion; it will only lead to someone "eating" your money. (The dating dynamic is one I return to in chapter 5.) Abstinence is an alternative choice, one that can save you money and make you more focused on your schoolwork, and this is no doubt an argument that resonated with youth (especially young men) so critical of the financial burden that sexual relationships created.

While abandoning sexual relationships had its financial and emotional appeal—no one wanted to feel he or she had been "used" by a partner—this alone could not account for why so many youth wholeheartedly embraced the message of clergy. Sexual relationships still brought students—especially young men—a significant degree of social status, and sex and intimacy were physically desired by many youth. The response of abstinence advocates was that the struggle to abstain had its own rewards that were evidenced in the mental and embodied transformations for youth that made them better, more successful people in the long run.

In church discussions of abstinence, the terms *accountability* and *intentionality* were earnestly used to demarcate this new sort of Ugandan youth culture, one more capable of managing and policing young people's desires and needs to create more efficient, self-sustaining citizens. Perhaps more than any other message, this one resonated with youth who were struggling to make their way in a city that frequently frustrated them. A member of UHC, Richard, emphasized the sort of distinction that abstinence and born-again spirituality brought youth when he described his peers who had not chosen the same path: "[Other people] cannot choose what to do and not to do, where to go and not. The reason is that they do not have the capacity to decide. They are not empowered. And for that reason they need information for empowerment, and that is what we try to do." Learning about and practicing abstinence was believed to empower youth; from their perspective it was a lesson that emphasized their own ability to control a certain part of their destiny. In particular, abstinence was a method through which young people could learn to channel and manage their desires—sexual and otherwise. It is

"Abstinence Is for Me, How about You?"

hard to overestimate the appeal of such a message. Richard explained to me in a series of conversations that he felt that many in his generation had been "lost," a term that resonates within born-again Christian circles because it implies those who have not been "saved" through conversion. But in his choice of this term Richard is also criticizing the attitudes of his generation. His peers are lost because they have no direction, no focus. They were "too free" in their embrace of the new liberties available to youth once they arrived in the city and on campus.

Another young man, Gideon, also spoke eloquently of the changes he felt abstinence had made in him. I met Gideon when he was a twenty-two-year-old student at the university; he had become involved in UHC through his interest in the church's newspaper. He was a charismatic and gifted young man who was especially interested in writing and expressed himself eloquently on his own blog, which he maintained for several years and which focused on Christian youth issues. When I last interviewed him, he was twenty-seven, had graduated, and was planning to get married. Explaining the sort of transformation that he believed abstinence enabled, he said, "What I have learned about sexual purity, it is character. It's more than dos and don'ts. It's the development of character. And it reflects so many other things. Of course, it is my faith. But the most important thing I've learned is that abstinence is character. You are building character to stay faithful to your future wife." Abstinence was believed to cultivate focus and drive; it made youth more "intentional" in their actions. As Gideon later explained, "Abstinence, it changes your mind. I know my mind is different because I have abstained." Here he emphasized the sense of self-transformation that the practice of abstinence was believed to cultivate. Youth felt that they were more in "control" of not only their sexuality but other actions and choices in their lives. Such control allowed them to be more productive, more invested in their decisions.

This sense of control and intentionality was never more important than when young people spoke of abstinence's effect on their relationships with other people. *Intentionality* was a term that was also used to emphasize the ways that abstinence allowed them to better choose whom they interacted with, whom they would eventually marry, and what that relationship would be like. They spoke about other people being driven by emotion, need, or obligation (which were perceived as negative qualities) rather than by reason. Abstinence allowed reflection on one's relationships and contemplation about the future of those relationships. Gideon explained how the new sense of responsibility that came with the practice of abstinence changed how he viewed his own current and future family relationships:

> I have been in one of those things, in a relationship that is not heading anywhere. You go out and you end up in some undefined thing. The church has prepared me by teaching me to be intentional. To be intentional in my relationships. It is not just "I love you, I love you"—so what? I can now work, knowing I am working to save money for my wedding, for my next stage of life. A family man, a person of values, a person who wants to mentor their children so they grow up not like I grew up. To be a cycle breaker. Those are very dear values to me. So the church has given me that commitment and that intentionality in being a man. That's what lacks most of all in men my age. There is no willingness to commit.

Abstinence was presumed to bring direction and decision making to the fore. Youth were told to plan for their relationships, to consider their options, and to enter into a "courtship" after serious deliberation. To abstain meant that youth worked to make themselves more accountable to those around them, more intentional in their relationships, and more calculating and rational in their plans for their own future. As I have noted, these traits were formed as part of a critique of an urban environment that was characterized by both temptation and frustration.

"Unintentional" Relationships: Criticisms of Traditional Family Life

A key difference that young people articulated between the lessons about sexual discipline associated with the home and the church's lesson about abstinence was that Christian abstinence taught them that control of their sexual behavior must come from within themselves rather than from external cultural or parental rules. Within the church abstinence was characterized as part of the larger pursuit of self-knowledge, the understanding of one's own desires, gifts, and flaws; this would in turn enable one to be more successful in life. Such self-reflection allowed youth to emphasize their independence from kin-based roles and obligations. Their place in society, the church emphasized, must come from "God's plan" for them; their social worth was not a function of their relationships within a kinship and clan system. Despite the criticisms levied at "traditional" values within the church, youth regularly sought to use practices of self-knowledge to reinvest in the traditional relationships of the family. Abstinence was not a way to withdraw from traditional ideas about moral behavior but a way of reimagining what tradition should be.

Esther was a typical member of UHC. Her childhood household was nominally Christian, and she did not become born again until she came to Makerere University, where she became actively involved at UHC. She had been raised in western Uganda by parents who spent most of their time living separately, in two different villages where they pursued their own separate business ventures. The separation was, in Esther's view, for economic reasons and with the intention of strengthening her family's status and economic stability. But her parents' decision to live separately was indicative of what Esther felt were larger social problems in Uganda, where traditional values often placed status or economic pursuit above the stability of the immediate family unit. This was a critique of tradition that was separate from the spiritualist critiques that were also common in this and many other Ugandan churches. (I will return to these critiques in chapter 4.) While traditional ritual and religious life was viewed as spiritually dangerous, Esther and her peers also felt that the traditional household was socially unfit. The rules of that household—rules of respect and deference to one's parents, rules that dictated obedience to authority—were characterized as "unthinking" by many of the youth I interviewed; they argued that such rules had been unsuccessful in crafting modern moral persons. Esther explained the differences between the regimented life of home and the sort of reflexive discipline that the church demanded (and which she preferred):

> I had the mentality [as a child] that you have to work hard in order to be okay in life. Now, in this other new family [of the church], it's about what God would want you to do. You might not work hard so much; or you might work hard but in the area where God would want you to be. They are two contrasting things. Back home, I knew you had to work hard. Whether you are at school, you need to read hard, go to discussion [study] groups. If you're at home, work hard for you to be okay. But here in church, life is quite different. I understand that we are gifted differently. And it's about the will of God.

Esther pointed out that her parents raised her to respect them and the rules of her home and school. She was taught to "work hard," to pass exams, and to pursue the degrees that are the markers of status and achievement. But she felt unfulfilled by these achievements. And she felt that the discipline of her household had clouded true understanding of her as an individual, with gifts that made her "special" and "unique" in the eyes of God. Her views were shaped in part by her position at the time of this interview: she had recently finished a degree in library science, a subject chosen because that was the one course for which she had been granted a seat at the university. But she did not like the work and could not, for that matter, find a job as a librarian in Uganda. She wanted to be a counselor, perhaps working with children, and thought she should pursue that career path instead. Like many of her peers—especially those who had finished their university education and were looking for work—there was a sense that the path that had been set for them held little in the way of fulfillment or promise. It was a path defined by the disciplinary structures of home and school, but one that had little to do with their own hopes and dreams. And it was a path that left Esther with little in the end but a certificate that held nominal value. The church, on the other hand, preached the optimistic message that youth should learn more about themselves and seek out ways to find career fulfillment even if it meant changing courses midstream or disobeying the wishes of elders. Esther explained that she felt that the church "family" was also disciplined, but it was a discipline that sought to shape her as her own uniquely gifted person.

A similar line of criticism argued that family disciplinary practices were "unloving" and opposed to the productive, loving relationships developed with God's help. A church parenting class I attended focused on discipline, and I remarked on how obedient and well-behaved Ugandan children usually seemed. The participants scoffed. "They are beaten!" several of them exclaimed. One woman said, "There is no love relationship between parents and children. Children aren't taught to understand their mistakes, only to avoid repeating them. This is because children are not considered real people." Another added, "They are ignored, mostly." For church members such discipline was characterized as mindless, and it was opposed to the mindful, self-reflective form of discipline that the church advocated. As Esther noted above, she was taught in church to understand her personal "God-given" gifts. She was told to learn her own passions and skills so that she could better actualize these gifts in the world. Such "self-knowing" practices were repeatedly emphasized at UHC. During a youth fashion show at the church the theme was "know your brand," an intentional co-opting of marketing lingo meant to emphasize young people's agency in their own self-making. If women could cultivate their own sense of style, perhaps they might also cultivate a better sense of who they were inside. And this sense of self, this process of self-actualization, was repeatedly contrasted with the regimented discipline of the traditional family.

"Abstinence Is for Me, How about You?"

Discipline and *self-control*, in the broadest sense of these terms, were key features of both traditional and church-based lessons about sexual behavior, but abstinence was interpreted as more appealing because it was related to a broader discourse of self-development, the cultivation of what church members called self-knowledge. Such discourse mimicked popular ways of speaking about economic development and social change in Kampala more generally. The neoliberal emphasis on individual choice and desire as a basis for broader social action and change was infused into many ways of thinking about society and self in Kampala. If you "knew yourself better" you might be better able to control your unruly desires, and you might be also better able to cultivate your skills and passions, become better educated, and find a more fulfilling job. Abstinence in this new global sense was not merely a moral discourse predicated on the maintenance of kin relationships and external obligations but was concerned with the development of a personal sense of spiritual and emotional sincerity.

Abstinence thus became a method for youth to criticize traditional morality and to assert a different way of being that they argued was superior. But abstaining was not simply a rejection of ideas about being a "respectable" person that had defined older models for moral behavior. These young people wanted to use abstinence to repair relationships, not abandon them. The questions of the participants at the church parenting seminar were common ones both within the church and in Kampala: What has rapid urbanization and social change done to traditional families? What is the experience of traditional culture like today? The answers were often negative: women were "liberated" to leave children with maids and enter a corporate workplace; couples in cities delayed marriage because of its cost. From this perspective abstinence was viewed not necessarily as an embrace of Christian neoliberal values that were opposed to tradition but as providing young people a way to reassert a particular notion of what tradition should be.

Discussions of intentional relationships were used to engage models for traditional relationships, just as the same language had been used to critique contemporary intimate relationships. Gideon's plan to wed saw marriage much as it was imagined through an older lens: the building of an affinal relationship marked the acquisition of a new social status. In this sense abstaining was experienced not as a withdrawal from relationships but as a better "management" of them. Anne, a young woman held in high esteem by her peers (in part because she was married to one of the lay leaders of the church), also emphasized how her thinking about relationships had been changed by church teachings. She believed that relationships required a certain amount of calculating reflection, shepherded by God's guidance:

> Also, I have learned about relationships. Before I got married, how do I know that this is the right person? How do I do that? In [the women's prayer group] you are taught to be deep with God. You have to know God, in that you actually know him and have a relationship. When you come to a point of making decisions in your life, God helps you. You do not just fall into a relationship. You are not like, "I have just fallen in love with this person, I am head over heels with him." No. What comes first? God comes first. And you are able to sort out things. That is what was very basic with me in finding my husband. Being informed.

For many young people this was an intensely appealing message; the framework of self-knowing and intentional relationships allowed for a reassertion of certain interpretations of traditional values while also emphasizing youth autonomy and agency. Self-critique, self-improvement, and autonomy were developed as skills that were channeled back into improved familial and social relationships.

To be intentional in one's relationships was meant as a direct criticism of the relationships that youth did not choose—relationships of obligation that defined their dependence on and responsibility to their families, clans, and kin groups. The messages of the church that focused on knowing oneself, planning for the future, and understanding one's own gifts and emotional temperament played off the frustration with family life that demanded obedience but did not guarantee—especially in the contemporary era—social advancement or success. Young people often had fraught relationships with their parents and other family members. Parents were viewed critically within the church, so much so that church leaders felt that young adults needed to attend the "parenting class" mentioned earlier before they themselves had children. The class emphasized how parenting in a "Christian way" was different from traditional parenting styles;[31] discipline was defined as a "restoration" of the family fellowship after a child's transgression. The emphasis was on the sincerity of a child's confession and how children must learn not only regret but also repentance. The class attendees found this lesson revealing because they believed typical Ugandan disciplinary practices lacked emotion and sincerity on the part of both parent and child. The woman of the pastoral couple leading the class reminded the group of a common saying: "Can a

"Abstinence Is for Me, How about You?"

parent go wrong?" It was a rhetorical problem repeatedly posed to children who questioned a parent's decision or actions. She explained that in a traditional Ganda household parental discipline was unreflective and insincere, requiring little empathy. The idea was that such discipline maintained and asserted the hierarchical relationship between parent and child rather than cultivate the view that parenting involved the fostering of a child's individual Christian moral compass. Here the family was viewed as a bulwark against immoral behavior, as a necessary part of young people's moral development. But youth were taught that the experiences of moral decision making and the nature of moral relationships were different in a Christian household from how they were in a traditional Ganda one.

Abstinence was a moral discourse that encouraged youth to imagine different ways of being "respectable" people. The idea of intentionality in relationships set abstinence apart from other moral paths; it was a discourse and a practice that emphasized youth agency and choice in relationships, but it also recognized young people's ambiguous feelings about family obligation, their desire not to abandon such ties but to reformulate them. In short, abstaining youth sought to restore—but also better control—their relationships with families by adopting a moral discourse that brought them status through its distinction. The practice of abstinence, like the work of Christian parenting, necessitated that they reimagine moral dilemmas as problems that were internalized, challenges that encouraged them to cultivate themselves as better Christian persons with "sincere" feelings. This process was opposed to the ways youth characterized moral choice in the scheme of the traditional family, where obedience—rather than reflection—was believed to be the most prized trait. Youth further extrapolated from these lessons the idea that the cultivation of the traits of self-knowledge that Christian abstinence required made them better, more "flexible" citizens, well suited to the vagaries of getting by in contemporary Kampala.[32] If you knew yourself better, if you understood your weaknesses and your desires, your strengths and "gifts," you were better suited to navigate a city where a job was far from secure and where *adaptability* and the *entrepreneurial spirit* were code words for success.

Conclusion: The Limits of Choice, Intentionality, and Accountability

The Kampala youth I knew attempted to reframe abstinence in terms of a shifting moral terrain that was especially complicated by the historical realities of the neoliberal city. Abstinence was for them a way of commenting on and reasserting new ideas about moral behavior given a social landscape that was fraught with many dilemmas related to sexuality. It was a message that was deeply mired in the language of neoliberal reform—accountability, self-sufficiency, personal empowerment—but in its practice youth used this language to express misgivings about values like personal freedom, which they associated with misguided, "lost" youth. Rather than simply embracing an American message about sexual self-control, these young people talked about abstinence in a way that reflected diverse models for sexual and moral behavior and different attitudes about what sex might ideally be.

The billboard I mentioned at the beginning of this chapter asked, ABSTINENCE IS FOR ME, HOW ABOUT YOU? In the early years of the twenty-first century, abstinence in Kampala was framed as a strategy for upward mobility, a way to gain status and become more successful. This was meant to be an aspirational message, inspiring youth to be "better." But with its pictures of book-carrying youth the billboard also signaled a message that established the choice to abstain as one that belonged only to a certain type of person. The language used to describe abstinence in Uganda clearly flagged it as an elite behavior—from the billboard that emphasized educational success to the church that emphasized planning and self-sufficiency. Abstinence was a practice that marked youth as different, as set apart from ordinary Ugandans, and as a class of people familiar with the discourses and techniques of the self associated with neoliberal modernity.

What I have not discussed at length in this chapter is how abstinence was a mode of self-actualization demanding that youth already occupy a position of relative privilege in society. To make the "choice" to plan for one's sexual partners assumes that an individual is the only factor that contributes to that decision, but in reality such choices demanded that youth be largely freed from immediate economic demands and that young women, in particular, feel socially capable of refusing sexual advances from more powerful male suitors. This was a discourse about sex that made many assumptions about the relative equality of men and women but disregarded the role that material support plays in intimate relationships in Uganda—topics I will explore in chapter 5. Predominantly schoolgoers, the young people I knew were largely supported by their extended family and felt only limited pressure to contribute economically to their natal household. And as university students—even though they were not all members of Uganda's elite—they had financial and social resources available to them that made sustaining their sexual decisions easier.

I am often asked whether the youth of UHC actually did abstain. For all the talk of sexual purity, did they follow through and remain sexually chaste? I did not collect data that tracked compliance with this message (it would have been difficult to collect accurate information within a community where admitting a failure to abstain had serious consequences), so my observations are anecdotal. Compliance within the church community, among the inner core of a congregation for whom the church was a primary social force, appeared to be high. There were few rumors about illicit sexual behavior, and there was a great deal of emphasis placed on the surveillance of peers. Intimacy between members of the opposite sex was strictly forbidden, and one-on-one socializing between men and women was strongly discouraged. This is not to say that everyone was abstinent, but it was unlikely that active members of the community could have regularly broken a pledge of abstinence without it becoming public knowledge. This points to the role that the community itself played in the practice of abstinence. Like others who have studied AIDS prevention within Christian communities in Africa,[33] I found that community surveillance played an outsized role in ensuring the feasibility of abstinence and marital faithfulness as successful prevention strategies. Among the students active at UHC, the church was their primary community, one often referred to as a second family, and many members spent part of every day with other members of the church, often on church grounds. Breaking a pledge of abstinence within this group would have had serious social consequences, including expulsion from the church. A couple who went before the church congregation one Sunday to admit that they had failed in their pledge of abstinence before marriage were quietly encouraged to leave the church, even though they were in the process of planning their wedding—and were married within weeks of their confession. The message of abstinence was an appealing one within the larger university community, but compliance depended on belonging to a smaller group in which choices regarding intimate relationships were closely monitored and adherence to a pledge of abstinence was supported and enforced both socially and spiritually.

As youth moved forward with intimate relationships, for instance by entering into church-sanctioned marriages, this sense of community could also bring a false sense of security to young adults. Young people who belonged to the church were encouraged to think of themselves as a group set apart—"saved" both spiritually and physically. Such rhetoric could be problematic as couples transitioned from abstinence to a "faithful" marriage, where compliance depended not only on their own behavior but that of their partners. As I will discuss in chapter 5, the sole reliance on the message of abstinence and faithfulness could close off discussions of risk that existed not only outside the community but also within it.

I highlight these points because abstinence is often portrayed by its supporters, both in Uganda and the United States, as a foolproof prevention strategy, one that places the onus on the individual: if the "right" decisions are made, the individual will be "safe." But as I have outlined here, safety, success, and even moral behavior can be viewed from a number of perspectives. Abstinence was not merely a reiteration of an American perspective on sexual self-control; it was a discourse about sexual behavior that was used by both elders and youth in Uganda to comment on and engage with a set of over-lapping ideas and practices relating to sex. It became a way to reassert and also reframe ideas about traditional persons and obligations, freeing youth to pursue a model of "respectability" that differed from the one forwarded by their parents. This made abstinence deeply appealing, but it also may have limited the number of Ugandan youth who felt the message applied to them.

What is more disconcerting is an emphasis on choice and youth empowerment that doesn't acknowledge the ways young people's decisions are often circumscribed by other factors. In the abstinence movement in Uganda, the failure to abstain—and indeed one's potential infection with HIV—is framed solely as an individual failure. This emphasis on personal agency in matters relating to health and sex has the potential to influence the ways in which people attribute blame for the disease and may turn attention away from efforts that attempt to intervene in the structural factors that shape individuals' perspectives on risk and choice. I take up some of these complicated issues in subsequent chapters, and especially chapter 5, where youth decisions about and plans for romantic relationships are discussed.

4 ABSTINENCE AND THE HEALTHY BODY

Spiritual Frameworks for Health and Healing,
or "The Right Way to Live Long"

On Valentine's Day, 2007, about a year after I moved to Kampala to conduct fieldwork, I attended the daily lunchtime prayer meeting at University Hill Church (UHC). Young people sat on the rustic benches that ringed the walls, or paced across the weathered floorboards of the prayer shelter that sat behind the house that served as UHC's office building. That day there was a giddy anxiety in the air; the students were restless. In Kampala, Valentine's Day has become a major holiday for urban young people who find themselves drawn to participate in the mass consumption of romance: flower arrangements for sweethearts, dinners at rose-petal-strewn restaurants in town. While the embrace of Valentine's Day has been rapid in recent years, it has not been without controversy. Popular sentiment is strongly divided on the holiday, with many newspaper editorials and street commentators pointing out the gratuitous expense of "romantic" gestures, and others—often elders—highlighting how romantic attitudes seem to support a "culture of dating" that makes relationships dangerously dependent on the whims of young people's hearts. Yet most young people, for many of these same reasons, eye the trappings of Valentine's Day longingly.

As committed members of the church, nearly all the youth at this meeting had pledged to abstain from sexual activity before marriage, which left them mostly on the sidelines as their peers prepared for elaborate celebrations with romantic partners. In the church romance was not disavowed per se, but it was considered the purview of married couples. Courtship—the Christian alternative to dating—was a practice distinguished by its chaste distance from both sexual intimacy and capitalist consumption. As much as it was desired, participation in Valentine's Day activities was meant for others, a realization that clouded that day's prayers with an added sense of nervous tension driven by the prospect of (much) delayed gratification. As the group finished its meeting, Pastor Thomas Walusimbi appeared at the corner of the shelter and marched to the front to share his thoughts on these matters. Usually a boisterous presence, he cut an especially striking figure that day; he was wearing a white lab coat and dangling a shiny stethoscope around his neck. The assembled church members laughed, not knowing what to make of his new costume. He smiled broadly and proclaimed that his outfit reflected his authority as a "spiritual doctor"; he was there to help "cure" our problems. Abstinence, he went on to assure the group, was the solution to our ills and worries; it would lead us to our spiritual and economic emancipation. We needn't trouble ourselves over broken hearts and empty pocket books; abstinence would heal us. It would relieve our burdens.

For a song released that Valentine's Day that would soon be playing on Christian radio stations in town the pastor had teamed up with a popular gospel star. Their performance riffed on the pastor's new medical persona: the gospel artist introduced Walusimbi as "the doctor," and at a later concert featuring the pair the pastor was again sporting his borrowed hospital gear. Their song reminded listeners that abstinence and faithfulness were the paths to long, prosperous, and healthy lives. Marriage, created by God, was meant to join one man and one woman, giving them sanctuary in which they could protect each other and their children and in turn "build the nation." In the chorus they sing, in Luganda:

Maama mugambe:	*Tell mama:*
bwesigwa bwe bukuuma amaka	*faithfulness, it protects the home*
Taata mugambe:	*Tell papa:*
bwesigwa bwe bukuwa eddembe	*faithfulness, it gives you peace*
Switihaati mugambe nti:	*Tell sweetheart:*
bwesigwa bwe bukuwangaaza	*faithfulness, it makes you live long*
Mu nsi eno bw'otaba,	*On this earth, if you are not already,*
mwesigwa, ekituufu tuwangaala	*be faithful, the right way to live long.*

As I discussed in chapter 3, abstinence (along with its fellow virtue, faithfulness) was a moral discourse about behavior. But it was also a practice that was believed to ensure health and well-being for its practitioners. It was a method by which youth were told they could secure their protection from AIDS and live long and healthy lives. Within the church abstinence was considered a spiritual practice, one shaped by other practices of healing and discourses of health and illness that existed alongside it. In particular, the

Abstinence and the Healthy Body

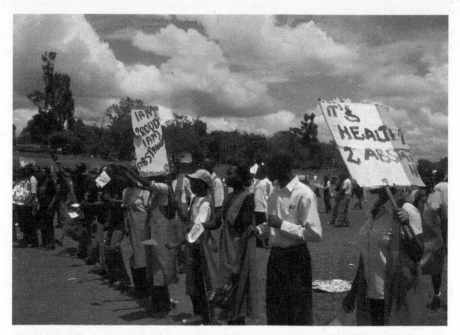

FIGURE 4.1. "It's healthy 2 abstain"; rally in support of abstinence, Kampala, October 2006

church emphasized the ways abstinence provided a method of spiritual protection of the self that was believed to be more effective than other paths to
healthiness in Uganda. Pastor Walusimbi's explicit effort to co-opt symbols
of medical technology spoke to how abstinence was framed in terms of the
broader context of biomedicine and to the ways youth viewed abstinence as
something different from—perhaps exceeding—the protective qualities offered solely through biomedical interventions. Walusimbi was a "spiritual
doctor": his demeanor, language, and symbolism outlined a healing power
that encompassed, and surpassed, sole reliance on the biomedical realm.

This chapter highlights how spiritual beliefs shape relationships to the
body in particular ways—ways that influence how people interpret and apply public health messages. Abstinence engaged the broader field of healing
and spirituality in Uganda, and intervened in local experiences of health and
disease. It was understood to be a method of ensuring health, a message championed by the placard waving young adults I witnessed at a proabstinence
event in Kampala in 2006 (see fig. 4.1). But what sort of health (spiritual, social, physical) did abstinence help define? Throughout this chapter, I consider the ways that Ugandan experiences of spirituality and health have given

shape to the practice of abstinence, and in particular to the ways abstinence was framed in the church as a spiritual practice with therapeutic power. I focus especially on the practice of deliverance prayer, through which youth are encouraged to contemplate their relationships and "cast out" those that are considered ungodly. This practice of spiritual reflection is understood in the church to be a spiritual extension of the physical practice of abstinence, one that reveals the ways that youth understand the relationship of their bodies, minds, and spirits. My discussion of youth abstinence engages a longer history of inquiries into the nature of healing in Africa, as well as more recent concerns over the role of Christianity in mediating the experience of contemporary health on the continent.

The Pursuit of Health in Uganda:
Interdependence and Moral Personhood

At first glance, the assertion that the experience of illness may vary across cultures goes against our own popular notions about the naturalness of physical experience: the intimate, personal, and perhaps especially noncultural realm of illness, biology, and health. Yet the variability in how people make sense of disease and its causes has formed the cornerstone of historical and anthropological studies of healing. In studies of Western medicine, anthropologists like Emily Martin have pointed out how American metaphors for illness—viewing the body as a "machine" or, later in the twentieth century, a "flexible system"—articulate particularly American cultural values and notions of the person, and especially the belief in the individual's capacity for transformation, self-discipline, and self-reliance.[1] Claire Wendland, in her insightful ethnography of a medical school in Malawi, has described biomedicine as a "moral order" that shapes the behavior and attitudes of student doctors. A medical doctor, for instance, is trained to think about her patient in particular ways; not as a product of a particular social community, living within certain cultural and economic constraints, but as an "autonomous— yet universalized—individual."[2] The work of Wendland, Martin, and others has demonstrated that the ways we think about, experience, and describe health—even in the rarified scientific realms of biomedical research and the technological maze of the Western hospital—are in part social orientations that are shaped culturally and historically.[3]

Ugandan and other African experiences of disease, illness, and well-being are not often expressed through the metaphors of physical containment and self-reliance familiar in the West. Anthropological studies of African health have focused attention on the ways that healing is often "fundamentally concerned with the reconstitution of physical, social, and spiritual order."[4] That is, in many African societies the pursuit of health is not limited to a focus on the individual body, but is often oriented outside the self. Healing practices seek to remediate illness by addressing the social and spiritual relationships that are believed to give shape to physical well-being. Neil Kodesh, whose historical study of clanship in Buganda considered the relationship between healing and political power in the kingdom, has argued that in Buganda people "perceive the pursuit of well-being as a collective endeavor."[5] Individual physical health and prosperity in Buganda were—and in many ways continue to be—understood as a function of the well-being of the extended clan, and illness and misfortune were traced and remedied by addressing one's relationships to others, both past (ancestral) and present.

Susan Reynolds Whyte's study of contemporary experiences of illness among the eastern Ugandan Nyole people similarly highlights how sickness is understood in that society as a function of one's social and spiritual relationships. Taking E. E. Evans-Pritchard's famous query, Whyte modifies it slightly: "[T]he question I hear Nyole people ask is not 'Why me?' but 'Why you?' Their immediate focus is not on the self, but on the other: who are you behind this affliction and why are you doing it?"[6] She notes that this mode of questioning focuses inquiries regarding suffering outside the self, requiring the afflicted to take into consideration the motives of other agents and to adjust therapeutic action accordingly; this forces moral reflection onto a broader network of relationships and kin. As in Buganda, ideas in Bunyole about health are tightly bound to experiences of the person, the body, and social identity that are especially relational and that emphasize an individual's social interdependence.[7]

Whyte's and Kodesh's longitudinal studies of healing in these two Ugandan societies point to the ways in which the pursuit of health and wellness demands moral reflection on the nature of the person and, especially, the relationship between the physical body and the social category of personhood.[8] It also necessitates consideration of the nature of misfortune and our obligations to those afflicted: How is the body itself imagined in moral and spiritual terms? How are physical problems reconciled in response to such orientations? As Whyte has eloquently noted, in asking these questions we are forced to reflect on the broader moral and social concerns that give such questions shape.[9] Who or what is to blame? Why are we the ones faced with this affliction?

The pursuit of health—whether in the West or in Africa—has always been entangled in these larger questions about who we are and how we should intervene in the problems that threaten such security. Julie Livingston has written in her evocative ethnography of debility in Botswana that change to our bodily state "triggers the imagination," forcing us to reflect on ourselves not only as vulnerable bodies but as certain types of persons.[10] In this chapter, I take up the analysis of abstinence in terms of these sorts of questions—questions that highlight how healing engages with a fundamental struggle over the meaning and experience of moral personhood. It is also a struggle shaped by competing narratives in contemporary Uganda that seek to define embodied health, disease, and personhood in distinct ways.

Abstinence, far from simply a Western discourse about self-control, was appealing to Ugandan youth because it was also a practice that enabled youth to engage and reflect on their social and spiritual relationships. As a pathway to health, abstinence provided multiple strategies for dealing with the uncertainty of life in the time of AIDS. As it was understood at UHC, it was a discourse that encompassed two seemingly contradictory frameworks for understanding disease and its prevention: the individual-focused language of containment and control familiar to biomedicine and the relational idioms of traditional health care. In its embrace of multiple models of therapy, the work of abstinence mirrored the pragmatic strategies of other Ugandans seeking to remedy the misfortunes of disease.[11] The youth I knew embraced the practices associated with Christian abstinence as modes of action in response to increasingly uncertain social, moral, and economic worlds. In many ways their efforts to do so played out in a spiritual realm that they believed gave shape to their embodied experience of health. It is to the spiritual realm, and its role in the pursuit of health, that I now turn.

Ugandan Spirituality and the Pursuit of Well-Being: Health of Body and Spirit

For born-again Christian youth, as for most Ugandans, the relationship between the spiritual world and the physical world was central to their experience of well-being. This is by no means a unique perspective on health; for most people worldwide, including many Americans, health is often expressed in terms related to a spiritual, nonphysical self. For many Christians the world over, the individual's spiritual relationship to Jesus provides the center around which the self—healthy, sick, troubled, or successful—is oriented.[12] Prayer in evangelical and Pentecostal churches often focuses on developing one's "personal relationship" with God, and it is through this relationship that a person learns to know and understand herself and to change her behaviors in ways that can influence well-being. This experience of the Christian self is one that Thomas Csordas illuminates in his study of charismatic healing in the United States; he writes that American charismatic healing does not concern specific "symptoms, psychiatric disorders, symbolic meaning, or social relationships."[13] Rather, the charismatic healers he observed worked to make the self "whole" again; their efforts were focused on addressing and mediating the break between sinfulness and righteousness that defines the Christian soul. Csordas argues that healing in these communities emphasizes an experience of personhood predicated on the articulation of spiritual and physical autonomy and a focus on interior transformation and personal agency. In short, these healing practices help orient and constitute a particular notion of the person that dominates, and in part defines, American Christian culture.

While American and Ugandan Christians share a concern with the interdependency of spiritual and physical health, the ways in which this relationship is imagined differ in significant ways. These differences shaped how Ugandan youth thought about and experienced their healthy bodies and the ways they envisioned threats to their well-being. This orientation to the body and spirit also shaped their understanding of and attraction to abstinence. As I describe in more detail below, Ugandan young people's experience of the Christian person, and the spiritual world that gives that person shape, was significantly influenced by a cultural framework that might best be described as relational and that differs from the pursuit of internalized "wholeness" that Csordas argues is central to American Christian approaches toward healing.

The Baganda and other Ugandans believe that their personal health is in part shaped by the status of the relationships they have with those around them, with those to whom they are related, and with those from whom they are descended. Illness and misfortune have long been addressed in Ugandan communities by relying on methods that seek to restore the moral order that defines relationships of mutual obligation within the lineage and clan—for example, by maintaining ancestral shrines or making offerings to appease spirits or gain their assistance. Seeking out the cause of an affliction demands reflection on this broader spiritual world, one where ancestral ghosts, human cursers, and other spiritual forces have direct influence on one's health. Modern efforts to heal are often refracted through this experience of collective well-being. Rather than rooting therapies in remedies shaped by abstract statistical or technological expertise, as is often the case in the biomedical realm, Ganda traditional healing integrates a focus on "establishing productive relationships with a variety of spiritual entities . . . [that anchor] the social health of communities."[14]

Even today, when most Ugandans rely on biomedical therapies (e.g., pharmaceuticals and surgery), one's well-being is still expressed, at least in part, as a function of a broader spectrum of social conditions and relationships—to one another, to one's ancestors, and to the environment. As compared to many Western cultures, and especially certain Christian traditions, a key difference is that the spirit is not understood to be a disembodied phenomenon set apart from—or, as it is the case in ascetic Christian thinking, in an antagonistic relationship with—the body (i.e., the soul must subdue the carnal will of the flesh).[15] In Buganda and Uganda more broadly, physical and material substances have spiritual significance and import, giving shape to the spirit and also making the body vulnerable to evil and the ill will of others. Similarly, the body does not contain or bind the spirit; the spirit extends beyond the body's limits and is traced in and through one's relationships to others in a dynamic fashion. This is an experience of the physical body that highlights its permeability and its vulnerability to both material and spiritual influences that may alter the nature of the person.

One example of this dynamic is found during *kwabya lumbe*, the Ganda succession ceremony that follows the end of a mourning period. During the ceremony a living successor is named to fill the place of the deceased in the lineage, taking on the practical obligations and responsibilities the deceased held in the family. Such ceremonies are notable for the ways they articulate an experience of the person shaped by the spiritual contingency of the body and soul, the ways an individual person comes into focus through a changing matrix of relationships of spiritual and material obligation. The ceremony creates a spiritual bond between the deceased and the named heir in such a way that the heir may physically "inherit" the personality traits of the departed—that is, the spiritual bond between the living and the dead may alter the living person's experience of self. A friend who had participated in one such ceremony and was named the spiritual heir to her great aunt described to me how in the years following the ceremony she sensed that her personality had changed, and she began to act more like her great aunt; this was a sign to her and her family that she had indeed "inherited" her great aunt's spirit. This ceremony is one example of the ways the physical body and person are believed to be dynamically shaped by spiritual relationships.

Abstinence and the Healthy Body

An heir makes a powerful promise, taking on the responsibilities of the deceased and inhabiting the lineage position of that person, with all the obligations and burdens that entails. Agreeing to take on such a responsibility establishes a spiritual relationship that many Baganda believe physically changes a person, altering his or her own sense of identity.

The act of naming carried similar concerns for the youth I knew. At UHC, members were taught to reflect on the meaning of their names and the sorts of spiritual ties and relationships such names created. In most of Uganda, children are given at least two names, one from the father's clan and the other a Christian or Muslim name, depending on the family's beliefs. For instance, Esther Nakimuli (sometimes written Nakimuli Esther) is a Christian woman (Esther) whose father is a Muganda from the Ffumbe clan. At UHC many wondered whether their names, especially their clan names, made them beholden to a set of beliefs they did not share. Names were believed to affect one's character and sense of self. And like heirs in the *kwabya lumbe* ceremony, young people worried that names could carry the character traits and spiritual problems of the ancestors they were named for. Because of these concerns it was a common practice for members of the church to rebaptize themselves with a new name, one that was stripped of the spiritual connections that many believed animated clan names and given names. One young woman explained to me her decision to change her name:

> I shared a name with my grandmother and I used to demonstrate her
> traits. Not settling down, being confused. And so [the pastor] told me
> that you need to change your name. So I took six months praying
> about it. And so I said, "God, tell me if I should change my names."
> In the Bible people are changing their names in line with a call upon
> their lives. One night I had a conviction in my spirit. And ever since I
> have changed my name my life has changed. Maybe it is just a mind-set.
> But ever since I have changed my name I have been able to complete
> things—start and finish things.

Those who changed their names emphasized to me the changed sense of self they experienced upon renaming. To take a new name was to sever the links to one's ancestor that were believed to create not only symbolic connections to one's past but physical and emotional ties that could directly affect bodily states.

This experience of physicality and selfhood generates intense reflection on personal and ancestral relationships when questions about health arise. This is not necessarily a unique orientation toward the body. As Julie Livingston points out, in the West "such intuitive notions float just under the surface of overt statements and beliefs about individually bounded bodies and Cartesian mind-body dichotomies."[16] But in Uganda, concerns about bodily vulnerability are often expressly linked to concerns animated by the sense that one's health is affected by one's physical and spiritual relationships. The overwhelming present-day concern with the practice of witchcraft in Kampala, and elsewhere in Africa, underscores the ways in which the status of one's relationships with others figures prominently in cosmologies of bodily well-being.

At UHC the danger of witchcraft was a frequent topic, one that was often used to elucidate the vulnerability of the body to spiritual assault. Gladys, a charismatic worship leader married to a junior pastor, told me on several occasions that she had long struggled with her father's new wife's use of witchcraft, a practice that Gladys believed to be socially and spiritually dangerous. After her father had remarried, Gladys learned that his new wife used witchcraft to ensure that her father would not take other lovers and that he would spend money the way she wished him to. More troublingly, Gladys's father had recently been ill, and Gladys now felt that this illness was also caused by his wife's use of witchcraft. Concerns about witchcraft are often conveyed to underscore the danger of unchecked self-interest, especially as such self-interest is expressed in terms of a spiritual/magical effort to control the behavior of others to one's own benefit. As other scholars have highlighted, such practices may point to tensions over personal conduct and social obligation, perhaps especially a sense of moral ambivalence about new forms of wealth, power, and inequality in modern society that challenge traditional notions of status and obligation.[17] In this sense, concerns about witchcraft reveal how physical health is understood as viscerally contingent on the maintenance of social obligations and the rightful investment in relationships of mutual obligation. Gladys believed that the new wife's self-interest, her abuse of this relationship, was manifested in Gladys's father's illness; his well-being was in part tied up in the agency and behavior of his wife.

Christian healing in Africa has usually taken these and other ideas about the spiritual realm seriously but has sought to assert a Christian spiritual authority that is superior to, and able to intervene in, the realm of ancestral spirits and the spiritual forces of witchcraft that are believed to influence individual health.[18] At UHC the ideas about disease and affliction I have traced above were widely held. Problems students experienced—especially emotional distress (anxiety, nightmares, and the like), but also specific health problems such as menstrual cramps, alcohol addiction, insomnia, infertility, and the stillbirth of a child—were attributed to afflictions caused by spiritual ties to others through lineage and kinship. Deliverance ceremonies—which I discuss in detail below—used prayer and "spiritual warfare" to cast out dangerous relationships and sever such ties. As much as these were Christian ceremonies that focused on the competing spiritual forces of good (God) and evil (Satan), such ceremonies also allowed for intense reflection on a wide range of spiritual and physical relationships, from ties to one's ancestors to the spiritual ties forged with living friends and family. Every relationship, past and present, was believed to create a spiritual link between people, and it was this extended array of relationships that born-again youth and their pastors considered responsible for their well-being. Esther was a UHC member who believed her brothers were cured of their alcoholism through her deliverance prayer. She explained to me, "Every physical relationship, it has consequences in the spiritual [world]." The reverse also held true: the spiritual world, and the relationships in it, could affect one's sense of well-being and health.

For the youth of UHC the most important way to maintain physical, spiritual, and mental health was to regularly reflect on the state of their relationships with others. In church they were reminded to consider past relationships and seek to understand the cause of their misfortune or their ill feelings in terms of those relationships. Problems were most often traced to a relationship that had become unsettled, either long in the past (such as ancestral relationships) or in the present (relationships with a jilted lover or an uncle who practiced witchcraft). Prayer was then used to sever or rectify the spiritual remains of these problematic social bonds. Illness in this context was related to one's behavior, but it was an interpretation that viewed bodily health in terms that were intensely shaped not only by individual choices but also by social relationships and the maintenance and management of one's obligations to others that gave those choices shape. That is, it was not so much a personal choice to eat too much that made one sick (though such behavior could do so) but that the personal motivation behind that behavior—the reasons you had acted as you did—were viewed as linked to the status of the relationships you had with those around you. Because of this, members of UHC believed that the ability to control oneself, including one's ability to abstain, required constant attention to the spiritual realm. Self-control was a bodily practice that required not only personal will but also acknowledgment of the ways one's will was in part shaped by the spiritual and physical relationships that gave rise to a person. The choice to abstain was thus maintained by turning not only inward to reflect on one's own sinful mistakes and desires but also outward to reflect on the nature of one's ties to others and the ways those ties influenced behavior and well-being. This was an orientation toward health and behavior that played upon tensions between traditional and Christian spirituality, highlighting an older emphasis on the role of spiritual interdependence in health while also asserting a method to manage and even control its continued influence on personal well-being.

The Spiritual Work of Well-Being: Deliverance

Deliverance prayer is practiced by Pentecostals and other charismatic Christians worldwide, but in many parts of Africa it has proven particularly attractive for the ways it engages a theology of "spiritual warfare" that recognizes the power of local spiritual agents and provides a means to address and counteract such power.[19] Pastors at UHC often focused on the practice of deliverance in their lessons, and a series of Bible study meetings I attended during the first months of 2007 focused specifically on teaching church members the methods by which to identify and fight non-Christian spiritual agents. As I will discuss in more detail later in this chapter, deliverance was particularly important to youth because it proved to be a means by which they could manage and reflect on interpersonal relationships. Youth found that this kind of spiritual reflection was a necessary part of the practice of abstinence. For youth, abstinence was more than an expression of will that removed them from temptation. It was a practice the required constant attention to one's relationships, including those that were "ungodly," and recognition of the physical and emotional impact that such relationships could have on one's well-being. Deliverance gave youth the means to intervene in these relationships and address those that were problematic.

Deliverance prayer is different from other forms of prayer and spiritual reflection in that it is specifically intended as a mode of identifying the influence of evil in one's life and providing the means to "deliver" one from it. In this sense it is often explained as a restorative, even healing, practice for Christians. Esther shared the views of many when she spoke of the transformations to her troubled brothers' behavior in terms of their being "cured" of alcoholism after she had participated in deliverance prayer. In many ways deliverance prayer parallels certain traditional Ugandan healing practices, such as divination, in that it provides a method by which to identify the cause of

Abstinence and the Healthy Body

illness or misfortune.[20] It is a form of prayer that focuses on locating spiritual "ties" that may be harming a person, making him or her sick or bringing unhappiness.

The focus on an interrelationship between the spiritual and physical person obviously mirrors older Ugandan models of personhood and health, but a key distinction is that deliverance prayer seeks not to restore a broader social order but to manage, mediate, and often "break" or discard relationships that are viewed as damaging to the individual. This practice seeks to intervene in a spiritual world that is believed to influence health and well-being, but such interventions are focused on separating the individual from social obligations and networks rather than restoring or strengthening such relationships.

At UHC, lessons about deliverance often began with warnings about the unseen influence of the spiritual world on one's health. Pastor Herman, who was considered to be a specialist in deliverance prayer, began one Bible study meeting by revealing that many members of his own family had struggled with infertility, a devastating problem that had the potential—especially for women—to seriously inhibit the lives of those afflicted. Throughout Uganda infertility is often associated with concerns about the spiritual relationships of lineage and their effects on health; the inability to conceive and raise a healthy child is often viewed as a problem with roots that extend beyond the individual, potentially revealing an issue within the family, lineage group, or clan.[21] Because of these associations Herman's story seemed especially fitting for a lesson about the spiritual roots of physical maladies. As we sat on benches lined up to face one corner of the prayer shelter, where he stood at a lectern, Pastor Herman explained how he had come to understand and address the problems with infertility plaguing his family. He told us he prayed to God, asking for help and assistance. He described how, after a period of intense prayer, the vision of a drum was revealed to him, one that he believed had belonged to his grandmother. Drumming, especially by women, is associated with spirit mediumship in Buganda, and Herman inferred its appearance in his prayers to signal his grandmother's ties to powerful non-Christian spiritual practices.[22] Herman told us that he believed that the drum had cursed his family—possibly because of the spiritual work his grandmother had used it for—and that the curse had been inherited through the generations, causing the widespread problems with fertility his relatives suffered. Outside the church such revelations are usually addressed by attempting to confront and mollify the curser (whether ancestor or other spirit) or by counteracting the cursing agent used by a living person. But within the church community members were taught to recognize the power of curses as the work of the devil and to call upon Jesus to help "break" any curses that might bring affliction. Pastor Herman's curse represented an unwanted tie to his grandmother; the curse originated with her actions, a promise that she had made to the spiritual world, and it was now affecting her descendants. Herman explained that breaking this or any curse required "setting your heart against the devil," praying earnestly for Jesus to first reveal and then sever the unwanted spiritual tie that binds the Christian person, causing sickness or misfortune.

Deliverance and the Physical and Spiritual Costs of Sexual Relationships

For the youth at UHC, deliverance prayer reinforced the idea that every relationship that a person has in the physical world is mirrored in a spiritual relationship, and that the spiritual relationship has physical effects that may extend into the future indefinitely, even after you have ended your worldly ties to that person. Members of UHC were regularly reminded that they needed to be aware of their ancestors' non-Christian pasts, which were shaped by a spiritual world that today's Christians believed to be dangerous; it was a world that could still influence and affect a descendant's health. But contemporary relationships could also impact well-being; thus they were often reminded of the physical problems that personal—and especially intimate—relationships could have upon one's health. Esther, who I came to know well over my years of fieldwork at UHC, spoke to me at length about deliverance prayer in our first interview in 2007. At the time, pastors had identified her as having spiritual gifts that made her especially well-suited to prayer and prophecy. She believed she had a special aptitude that allowed her—through dreams and other methods of revelation—to identify spiritual problems in her own and others' pasts. The identification of "ungodly" soul ties—the problematic spiritual traces of physical relationships—was a key part of deliverance. It was only by identifying such ties that one could address them and "break" them, thus restoring health. Esther told me of her own most meaningful experience with deliverance prayer, a time when she came to learn and accept that she had been sexually molested as a child.

Her revelation followed a typical pattern. She was struggling with a sense that she was languishing, unhappy at school and unable to excel in her studies or find contentment. Often people pursue deliverance prayer because they feel an overall sense of disquiet or of physical unease, sometimes related to a feeling that their own personalities or dispositions are preventing them from achieving success or happiness. Sometimes these problems are expressed in terms of emotional dissatisfaction; other times they are traced to behavioral issues or specific physical maladies, as in the case of Pastor Herman's infertility. Esther told me that after she arrived on the university campus she felt out of sorts and was unhappy and unable to concentrate on her studies. She felt that "something was holding me back." Through prayer Esther came to "see" and remember being sexually molested by an older man when she was a young child. And she describes how she was able to use prayer to break the ties that the molester still harbored within her. Such ties are dangerous even if they are unknown to you and are not of your own doing, she explained; they are the source of a wide range of problems, but are especially associated with personal misconduct (failing school, drinking too much) and they may also lead to ill health or depression. By identifying and breaking the tie that the molester had forged with her through this abusive relationship she was able to cure herself of the physical and mental malaise that troubled her. I quote her story at length because it is characteristic of the frank way that the UHC youth often spoke of deeply troubling pasts and because it provides details of how these youth came to understand deliverance prayer and apply it to such problems. Esther's story also contextualizes the way most youth experienced the embodied relationship between the physical and spiritual worlds, particularly as she elaborated the interconnections between the elements of body, soul, and spirit.

> When you begin deliverance, they teach you their teaching about
> deliverance so you can easily see what might be binding you. Now, in
> my case, I didn't know that when I was a child I was molested. I could
> hear my parents talk of it, but just in a hidden way. So one time I was
> in deliverance [prayer], and somehow God speaks and I got a vision, I
> saw the private parts of a human being. And I said, "What is this?" And
> I got to thinking that there must be something related to sexual sin in
> my past that is holding [me] back that [I] need to deal with. And God
> showed me that I was molested, really showed me what happened.
> Now, I was molested when I was very young, at around the age of two
> or three years. So I could see what had taken place, I could remember
> that they took me to the clinic; that I was bleeding. But I couldn't see.
> Maybe [I thought] it was kids [who] were playing such things. But

deliverance, for me, was when I got to know. God just said to me, "You were molested when you were still young. So you need to deal with that and forgive the people that did it so that you may be set free."

So I come back to the soul ties. So, when you are in a relationship your soul is related to the person that you are relating with, like the opposite sex. Now that is called an ungodly soul tie. If that relationship is ungodly, like if I am fornicating, that is an ungodly soul tie. So my soul is connected to your soul. Now, I am imagining that you are my boyfriend—our souls are connected such that sometimes I can even sleep and dream about you and sometimes I can even sleep and dream that we are having sex—such things.

I said that the body, the human being, is made up of three components: the body, the soul, and the spirit. Now, when I get a dream and I see myself fornicating with someone before I am married, that means that in the spirit world, our spirits, we are married. Because spirits are like air, really: they can easily travel when we are sleeping. So you can easily get a dream that you are fornicating with your boyfriend, you understand? So in deliverance you, before you go to deliverance, you can easily be getting these dreams. But you can test deliverance when you stop getting those dreams. During deliverance you confess of that sin, you renounce it, and then you release the people that did it, and then you forgive them. When you forgive them you begin dealing with covenants in the spirit world. You break covenants of spirit marriages, you break covenants of sexual fornication. It's like when you are praying in church to God, you don't see him but you are speaking to the spirit realm. "I cancel [renounce] this and this"; you are just praying. So even in confession you can say that you break that covenant that was made in the spirit realm, the spirit world: covenants of sexual immorality, of fornication. So there you are being set free. But you can really test your deliverance because you begin operating the proper way that God wants you to operate. You can know that you are set free when you don't struggle with these things again.

Esther's story outlines how relationships were believed to directly impact health. Their effect was considered to be much broader and less tangible than the physical traces of sex, or the conscious emotional bonds of love.

Physical relationships were believed to leave spiritual traces (soul ties), and these traces, whether known to one or not, could influence one's well-being. If a relationship was "ungodly"—because it was predicated on sinful behavior (fornication or sexual abuse), for instance—the youth at UHC expected that tie to generate a sense of unease or ill health within a person. These spiritual ties might also persist even after a relationship had physically ended. One might vow never to see a boyfriend or girlfriend again, but that relationship would continue to have a physical effect because of the enduring influence of a soul tie.

Esther explained that an important way one might learn of these effects was through the dreams one had about past relationships. Because of this, dreaming was viewed as an important diagnostic tool that UHC youth were taught to cultivate. It was a way to understand the state of one's spiritual health and identify factors that might bring harm. Dreams make one aware that a past relationship is "ungodly" and that it therefore must be accounted for and confessed, and then its spiritual ties severed. Without such interventions these relationships, like Esther's history of molestation, might continue to leave spiritual traces, traces that could harm physical and mental well-being.

For youth seeking to abstain, deliverance was an important tool that allowed them to understand the nature and power of physical temptation. If their dreams and conscious thoughts were dominated by the memories of a lover, tempting them to stray from their pledge of abstinence, that was a sign that the lover held a special spiritual power over them, a power that could impact their behavior and decision making. Deliverance provided the means to address and sever the spiritual ties of past relationships, counteracting the negative influence and temptation of these external actors. Even for youth without past lovers, like Esther, deliverance was a tool that allowed them to better understand their own temperaments, and enabled them to better predict and alter their behavior. Such spiritual attention to the ways external relationships influenced one's sense of self was a critical aspect of the effort to abstain.

Health and the Management of Spiritual Relationships

These lessons about deliverance were appealing to the UHC youth in a number of ways. First, deliverance was a practice that recognized the power of a spiritual world that was believed to exist beyond the church, a world that many viewed as significant but about which they held deeply ambivalent feelings. Common rituals that surrounded marriage, birth, and death demanded that born-again Christian youth return to their families and engage with that ancestral spiritual world. But they were taught in the church that such ceremonies could be dangerous, and that non-Christian spiritual worlds were repositories for evil, ungodly spirits. All youth I knew harbored deep misgivings about the spiritual component of certain cultural ceremonies. When Pastor Gideon, a charismatic young leader in the church, was planning his wedding he told me he chose to "resist" his grandmother's efforts to "give me a blessing with some demonic stuff." He explained that he feared the effects of a non-Christian blessing and worried that such a blessing might obligate him to ancestral spirits in ways he did not wish to be obligated. As Pastor Herman's lesson about his grandmother made clear, the UHC youth were taught that such spirits were ever-present and potentially powerful— yet dangerous—influences on their lives.

Given the push and pull of non-Christian spirituality—its danger, but also its recognized power and presence—deliverance prayer was an attractive practice because it provided a method to manage relationships with the spiritual world. Deliverance allowed youth to pursue and engage this tension rather than deny it. Frequent ceremonies that "cast out" ancestral spiritual influences reasserted the very presence of these influences in people's lives but also gave youth the sense that they had some ability to manage and control them.

These lessons came into clearer focus during another midweek prayer meeting when Pastor Walusimbi came to the front of the room and told us that we needed to spend some extra time praying for a fellow church member. James was a student at the university who had begun to struggle with exhaustion. He was tired all the time, falling asleep in his classes and generally feeling out of sorts. He turned to his pastors for help, seeking relief from his restless nights. The pastors had prayed with James, and their prayers over him soon became forceful. It was clear that James's spirit was struggling with something; most likely other spirits had made a claim to him, forging ties with his spirit while he slept. Deliverance prayer was often intense, especially if the spiritual ties that were identified proved difficult to break. That was the case with James, and the pastors prayed over him for more than twenty-four hours, struggling against a spiritual force that resisted their efforts to "release" James. Over the course of that day and night pastors determined that James was a descendant of Ganda royalty and that his ancestral spirits were "stealing" his spirit away during the night in order to force him to fulfill his ritual duties on the royal palace grounds. His ancestors were claiming their rights to James's spirit, requiring that instead he "work" for them at night. This explained James's exhaustion, his feeling that sleep brought little relief to him.

After he had shared this revelation with the larger group, Pastor Walusimbi called all people with "royal blood" to the center of the room.[23] We were asked to pray for those people because they were "being called by other forces" and becoming destabilized by "sacrifices and these things the ancestors did." Walusimbi reminded us that we all existed in the spiritual realm and that we were not always aware of what was happening to our spiritual selves; we might be "used for other things" unbeknownst to us. We had to be vigilant in identifying and understanding the spiritual claims on our souls that might make us weak, sick, or unhappy.

Youth struggled to seek a balance between an ancestral spirituality that in many ways still defined who they were as moral and social persons and a Christian spirituality that taught them to fear such spiritual obligations. Family ceremonies posed special problems—especially those that specifically sought to celebrate and reinforce a sense of interdependence and obligation between the living and their ancestors. Many youth feared such ceremonies because they were taught by pastors to see the reassertion of spiritual kin and lineage obligations as threats to the coherence and inviolability of the Christian person. Sarah, whose experiences during and after the Ganda *kwabya lumbe* (spiritual inheritance) ceremony I recounted above, elaborated these sentiments when she told me,

> Such ceremonies try to make you connected to things you don't understand. It's a spiritual thing. Why should we continue to suffer this thing created without our knowledge? We believe we are spirits in a body that can be controlled by God or the devil. The ancestral spirits represent past promises that we didn't have anything to do with. [I am] against any obligations that are not known to me, that make me suffer. It is not that I hate my great-granddad, but that his spirit made an agreement that I do not know about. Why should I suffer from this?

Spiritual succession ceremonies were deemed important because they restored social order by reaffirming lineage and clan relationships and the present world's connection and obligation to the past. But in doing so such ceremonies articulated an experience that highlights the spiritual permeability of the body and soul, one's dependence upon others, and the way an individual person is shaped by a changing matrix of relationships of spiritual and material obligation. As I noted above, the successor in the *kwabya lumbe* ceremony was thought to inherit not only the social obligations of the deceased but the spiritual obligations and personal traits of that person. This spiritual interdependence was viewed as especially threatening to Christians, for whom the autonomy of the Christian soul and sincerity of individual belief and action defined moral personhood and spiritual salvation. Sarah felt this conflict deeply.

Like other spiritual discourses in contemporary Kampala (perhaps especially those concerning witchcraft), the practice of deliverance seemed to be animated by a rising sense of ambivalence, a certain tension surrounding changing attitudes about family and the spiritual ties of kinship and lineage that gave such relationships of obligation shape. Deliverance was attractive because it played upon and helped engage these tensions in ways that recognized, but also sought distance from, the continued importance of non-Christian spiritual worlds to young people's lives.

Deliverance also proved appealing because it demanded that youth reflect upon their present-day personal relationships. In this way deliverance was a practice that enabled abstinence. It was the spiritual work that animated a promise to abstain. And it was only with the constant vigilance that deliverance demanded, the attention to personal relationships and their spiritual effects, that abstinence was believed to protect and provide for well-being. In church, youth were taught to identify the relationships that were troubling to them and to manage and sever the spiritual holds those relationships were believed to generate. This was empowering for young people new to intimate nonfamily relationships. Church members often shared with me their stories of unsuccessful romantic relationships and the sense of anger and betrayal that followed the unhappy breakup of an intimate relationship. (When UHC youth spoke openly with me about them, these relationships were almost always described as having occurred before joining the church.) Past sexual relationships were often remembered, by men and women alike, as troubling. Their dissatisfaction with such relationships extended beyond a recognition that they were considered sinful relationships. Youth often harbored feelings of resentment toward past lovers or (as was clear from Esther's story) to the fact that they had been the victims of unwanted or violent sexual encounters. Women and men both considered deliverance important because it enabled reflection on the pain or heartbreak that these unhappy relationships had caused. In its demand for intense reflection about personal intimacy and emotional ties to others, deliverance became a significant way to address their feelings about love and companionship.

As I mentioned at the beginning of this chapter, contemporary discourses surrounding youth romance in Kampala are centered on a particular ideal of love, one associated with new patterns of consumption and new models of household organization. These modes of affection were thought to differ from older models of love and marriage in part because couples were taught to think of their bonds as independent from the broader matrix of kin relationships that defined traditional marriage. But even as modern love and courtship distinguished new relationships from older ones, newer relationships seemed less stable and secure. Relationships—especially those that had occurred outside the church, before the youth had become "born again"—were often associated with unhappiness and miscommunication. These experiences left lasting impressions, and deliverance became a way to address these feelings and to confess and sever the physical and emotional influences of past intimate relationships on present lives.

Deliverance as a central part of church practice was significant because it outlined and reinforced the interrelationship between spirituality and health, but it did so while emphasizing the Christian person's agency in shaping and shepherding that relationship. A healthy body demanded that young men and women focus attention on the spiritual relationships that gave shape to their person and that they intervene and address such relationships. This was the spiritual work that mirrored the physical lessons about intentionality that I discussed in chapter 3. Deliverance provided youth the means to manage their lived relationships and the effects those relationships were thought to have spiritually, mentally, and physically.

Conclusion: Abstinence as a Path to Health

The young people of UHC imagined, experienced, and expressed a variety of ideas about health. While the pursuit of good health generally included nonspiritual practices, such as eating well and using biomedical therapies when one fell ill, health was also widely understood to be shaped by spiritual relationships. Being healthy demanded that attention be paid to the maintenance and management of a spiritual world that mirrored and mediated the physical world, even if that entailed efforts to control or cordon off the spiritual world's influence.

Given this understanding of Ugandan orientations to health, how was abstinence engaged as a practice that would ensure good health? For all of the ways it seemed to reflect a broadly modern and global outlook, one that was shaped by an economic discourse that privileged the accountable individual, at UHC abstinence was considered to be a practice that also engaged other models for health and moral action. And its appeal lay in its ability to combine coexistent, yet seemingly divergent, strategies for coping with illness. While abstinence was securely located within a discourse of self-control and self-discipline associated with biomedical practices of hygiene and disease prevention, it also engaged another, perhaps contradictory, discourse. In pastors' lessons abstinence was often set against and believed to be superior to purely biomedical methods for preventing disease. Youth and pastors vilified condom use, claiming the method was dangerously unreliable in HIV prevention. Pastor Walusimbi's "doctor" persona was used to emphasize this point. He was a "spiritual doctor" whose medicine—faith—was the true cure for one's ills.

Abstinence was appealing in part because it was considered *not* so heavily reliant on the individual and was thus thought to be less prone to failure. Students would often remind me that no one could really be trusted to use a condom correctly in the heat of the moment; one could never rely on technology alone. This was a criticism hammered home in the church's student newspaper and at the Saturday night rallies held on campus. The message was simple: Individual will fails when it is separated from the broader context of spiritual and social relationships that shape a person. Biomedical messages about getting tested for HIV, knowing one's serostatus, and practicing safe sex seemed hopelessly abstract in comparison to abstinence.

In contrast to biomedical prevention strategies, abstinence was viewed as a socially oriented method for dealing with disease prevention. It addressed young people's relationships—past, present, and future—and sought to rectify those that were considered problematic. Deliverance prayer was a spiritual practice that animated the physical choice of abstinence; in many ways it constituted the "work" of abstaining. The choice to abstain demanded constant assessment of one's feelings, thoughts, and desires. The youth at UHC were taught to understand and identify lustful feelings as the work of the devil and to identify and cast out such influences on a regular basis. Just as other ungodly spiritual forces were managed and controlled through prayer, abstinence also demanded such spiritual reflection. As Esther explained, "Most perversions are associated with the spirit of Jezebel. Promiscuity, sexual deviancy, we understand them because of the story from the Bible.[24] So when we pray, we pray through the spirit. We must attack spirits." Lust should be managed and controlled through prayer because it is a product—like other desires and feelings—of the state of one's spiritual relationships. Too much sexual desire, or sexual desire at the wrong time or for the wrong person, is a sign that something is amiss spiritually.

Abstinence, as these youth experienced it, took into consideration this broader spiritual context. Edward said that when he learned about abstinence in the church it finally made sense to him. "It's not just that you are trying to keep away from pregnancy or what[ever]. There are two pieces. When you give yourself away, you give something more than your body. You give your dreams, you expose yourself to all those things that come around." Abstinence addressed Edward and his peers' concerns about the power of sex and sexual relationships. The instability of youth romances, and perhaps especially the physical desire for sex, made sex seem dangerous to these youth, even out of control. Abstinence was not just a message about saying no to sex. At UHC it fit securely into a broader spiritual struggle to make sense of changing values and relationship dynamics in contemporary Kampala.

Perhaps most fundamentally, abstinence strongly emphasized not only spiritual reflection but reflection on one's place within society and one's social relationships, recognizing not only the security of these bonds but also the ways they are frequently problematic and troublesome. Abstinence was experienced as a practical message for youth, one that spoke to the insecurities they felt about their future and their families. Alongside an emphasis on Christian marriage, abstinence was meant to provide youth with realistic and effective strategies for managing such kinship obligations. Within this community of young people this may have been its greatest appeal. Abstinence was, at its best, a strategy for managing relationships with others and for planning and securing future relationships (such as a formal marriage) that would bring new forms of status and security.

Many factors influence decision making as regards sex. The choice to abstain was one shaped by numerous constraints: financial, social, and spiritual. It was interpreted and made sense of within the broader context of health and embodiment in Kampala. Such contextualization allows us to understand youth motivations more fully, but it does not provide a predictive model for youth behavior. Nonetheless, a better grasp on the ways youth make sense of prevention messages is necessary if we are to understand how they interpret choices, risks, and incentives when it comes to sex. In the UHC community, spirituality was central to how youth imagined themselves as sexual persons, and their frameworks for spiritual and physical health differed considerably from Euro-American Christian models for bodily well-being. Abstinence emphasized spiritual agency and directly addressed spiritual and material tensions that shaped young people's relationships with their families. Given this it is likely that abstinence is significantly more successful as an HIV prevention strategy inside the church community than it is outside it—in Kampala and elsewhere. These limitations are significant because they make the promotion of abstinence to the exclusion of other messages about sexual health especially problematic in larger, more diverse communities. I take up some of these issues in more detail in chapter 5, which discusses young people's sexual relationships and attitudes about marriage in Kampala.

5 FAITHFULNESS
Urban Sexuality and the Moral Dilemmas of Love

For both its American and Ugandan advocates, abstinence was a message that seemed deceptively simple in its claim that self-control could protect young people from the risks of HIV/AIDS. But faithfulness was more evocative and poetic; this was a promise that sexual partners made to each other, not to themselves. It was a disease prevention strategy that depended not only on your personal will but on another person's dedication to you. In part because of this, criticisms of the promotion of faithfulness as a disease prevention strategy have been wide ranging. Scholars have pointed out that the message is linked, at least to some degree, to Western ideal models of marriage that seem out of touch in societies where the small, self-sufficient, and monogamous family unit is hardly the norm.[1] Other scholars have questioned the emphasis on faithfulness in societies in which ideal masculinity may be closely associated with the pursuit and support of multiple sexual partners and where a woman's right to resist the sexual advances of her (possibly unfaithful) husband may be legally and socially limited.[2] For these and other reasons, in societies around the world marriage has been correlated to a woman's *increased* risk for contracting HIV.[3] A health prevention message of faithfulness, its critics point out, obscures culturally variable sexual attitudes and norms and masks the political economy of sex itself.

Despite these criticisms, born-again Christian churches in Kampala embraced the U.S. President's Emergency Plan for AIDS Relief's (PEPFAR) emphasis on faithfulness and claimed it as a strategy that could control the spread of HIV and protect families and couples from infection. Well-versed in the arguments against this approach, pastors were particularly incensed by data linking marriage to heightened HIV risk. In a speech to his congregation in 2007, Pastor Thomas Walusimbi proclaimed "Marriage is the solution, not the problem! Marriage doesn't *cause* AIDS!" On World AIDS Day in 2006, born-again youth introduced a flag to promote faithfulness that depicted marriage as two gold rings, linked together and superimposed on a map of

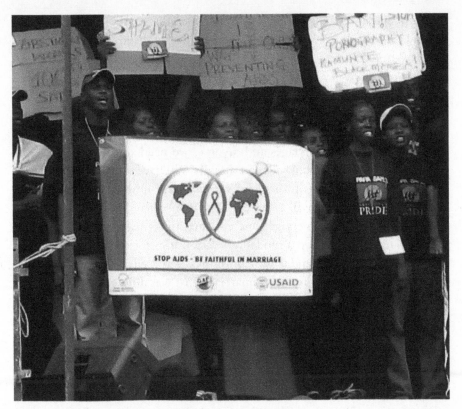

FIGURE 5.1. Faithfulness flag, Kampala, World AIDS Day 2006

the world, enveloped by a red AIDS awareness ribbon (see figure 5.1). Their message was clear for all to see: a "ring marriage"—long a euphemism for Christian unions in Uganda—was a safeguard against AIDS. Christian marriage was idealized, spoken of frequently in sermons, and planned for in church meetings and prayer groups. The hazards of contemporary sexual and marital relationships were acknowledged in church but viewed as problems outside the bounds of "faithful" Christian relationships. According to church leaders, gender-based violence, the economic migration that separates families, and the incidence of "sugar daddy" relationships between wealthy older men and younger women—all issues that contributed to the HIV risks of married men and women in Uganda—were not problems with marriage per se but problems that extended from a lack of faithfulness in family life.

For Christian youth, faithfulness was not simply a behavioral choice; it was a model for a new type of idealized marriage and family unit. For these young people it seemed a hopeful promise, one that could strengthen families and redeem "love" as the bond that cemented husbands to wives and parents to children, protecting them from sinful transgressions. Roberta, a member of University Hill Church (UHC), explained to me how abstinence leads to faithfulness and how faithfulness would then help foster love. "There is a better way to grow love, a better way to test love," she said. "If there is a way to kill HIV/AIDS as it spreads through the world, it is abstinence. . . . To avoid the broken marriages and divorce, we need abstinence. Because I have waited for you, waited *with* you, I really will have to spend my life with you. I will want to be faithful. And we will have healthy kids and have a healthy generation that will grow up." For Roberta and her peers, faithfulness was an optimistic message, one couched in terms of generational and social change. It described a model of relationships for the future rooted in an ideal of commitment and trust. Faithfulness was used to distinguish a new, supposedly more loving, model of marriage that was different from the partnerships of both "traditional" parents and contemporary peers. For born-again Christian youth, love was a transformative emotion, one that would rectify the problems of divorce, domestic violence, and infidelity; it was a shared sentiment that would change behaviors and in turn provide the groundwork for a new model of family life.

In part, this was a position grounded in a Christian faith in the transformative powers of love. Love, like the compassionate sentiment that animated American development projects discussed in chapter 1, was believed to create a bond between giver and receiver, one that would change both parties for the better. In the realm of such development projects, to show compassion was to share God's love, which in turn effected positive changes in recipients who received such care. Similarly, relationships of familial and romantic love were viewed as extensions of an individual's relationship to God; love was an emotion that originated in the experience of faith itself. Love, like faith, transformed people.[4] In Uganda, this Christian ideal of transformative love was experienced alongside other models for loving relationships and other ideas about the nature of the bonds between two members of a couple and among family members. In particular, faithful love was used to depict an image of an emotionally genuine, insulated, and self-sufficient couple, one whose love could shut out not only temptation but the social bonds and extended family ties that defined family life for most Ugandans. Christian love was portrayed as "sincere," a bond that was contrasted with both traditional family models and the popular ideal of romantic love that dominated youth culture in Kampala.

Christian Ugandans' embrace of the concept of faithfulness speaks to the importance of understanding how public health messages engage local discourses about love and other emotions. Attitudes about love were revealing of the ways young people at UHC considered and idealized certain relationships and evaluated the social worth and risk of various forms of intimacy. In this chapter, I examine how and why this message was taken up by Ugandans and put to use in Christian prevention programs. Faithfulness evoked ideals of a certain type of romantic love and was used to describe a model for marriage based on faith and companionship that in Ugandan discourse was opposed to other models for sexual relationships, both traditional and modern. Faithful love was a critical resource through which youth described their fears and desires for intimacy and companionship; it was a model that provided a way to scrutinize both the supposedly "loveless" marriages of their parents and the "lustful" pursuits of their peers. Their ideas about love also spoke to the problems they faced in pursuing intimacy and their opinions about ideal models for gendered and generational comportment. Understanding such affective dispositions and discourses about emotion are critical to our broader understanding of Ugandan sexuality, experiences of intimacy and desire, and evaluations of sexual risk.

Love and Health

Public health policies that advocate faithfulness highlight the moral and affective aspects of decision making as it regards behavior and health. Yet, in studies of disease prevention, love has been an overlooked emotion underlying behavior modification. Fear has been the most scrutinized emotional motivator for behavior change, and it is the sentiment most popularly associated with public health campaigns;[5] AIDS prevention programs in particular have long relied on fear to motivate change in populations. Ugandans who are old enough to remember them describe early prevention campaigns that focused on fear-based awareness—billboards ominously depicting the risk of HIV with the image of a skull and crossbones, and the regular broadcast of a "warning drum" signaling danger on national radio in the 1980s and 1990s. Studies of the emotional registers associated with public health campaigns have examined not only fear but also the emotional experience of risk and the feeling of disgust.[6] Love, when it is addressed, is usually highlighted as a problematic basis for a disease prevention message, especially that of sexually transmitted disease. Love may give individuals a false sense of security in long-term sexual relationships while undermining the pursuit of safeguards like the promotion of condom use within established partnerships or the regular HIV testing of sexually active couples.[7] The Ugandan slogan "Love Carefully," promoted by the government in the 1990s, has been especially scrutinized for the ways it gave couples a false sense of security; it seemed to imply that if you were "careful" in choosing a partner (by choosing apparently healthy-looking partners, or by simply loving your partner), your risk was negligible.[8] Researchers have rightly highlighted the structural risks associated with marriage and other long-term partnerships, but they rarely take on an analysis of love itself as a critical component of local forms of intimacy and how emotion plays a part in the ways relationships are pursued and evaluated as risky or safe.

Love may be ignored as an object of study for other reasons as well. Outside of a few fields, such as psychology, love has until recently been largely neglected as a subject of serious consideration.[9] Catherine Lutz, in her study of emotions in a Pacific Islander society, has described how in the West emotions are associated with the "ineffable" and with "devalued aspects of the world—the irrational, the uncontrollable, the vulnerable, the female," thus causing them to appear to lie outside the realm of serious scientific consideration. Moreover, throughout much of the twentieth century, emotions like love were considered to be individual, even biological, manifestations rather than shared aspects of social life that varied across cultures.[10] It is only in recent decades that scholars have acknowledged the importance of emotion to the study of social behavior and social change—and especially the ways emotional registers both shape and reflect variable cultural attitudes about sex and the nature of relationships between women and men.[11] While all humans have the capacity to love, "there is no universal, ahistorical experience of romantic love that all humans share."[12] Love, like all emotions, comes into being as a social and discursive practice, a shared sentiment that varies widely across cultures. Such variations contribute to how people within particular societies experience and pursue intimacy and companionship, and they are integral to any understanding of sexuality, family life, and marriage.

In the field of African studies, the initial scholarly silence on the topic of love has proved especially problematic. As Lynn Thomas and Jennifer Cole explain in the introduction to their volume *Love in Africa*, early researchers on the continent seemed to struggle to explain how "affective ties among Africans are present but different" from those in the West.[13] In societies such as Uganda's, love has long been expressed through practices of material support and care; it is an entanglement of love and money that challenges the Western view that emotions should exist apart from, and even opposed to, the material realm. The practice of bridewealth exchange throughout much of Africa appeared to Western observers as an affirmation that love was not the basis for marriages and family bonds. These assessments fed into long-standing racist depictions of African affect and sexuality, where libido rather than emotion formed the basis for sexual intimacy.[14] In AIDS research such assumptions fueled misguided early theories of how and why the epidemic spread so effectively on the continent.[15] Such work, in pursuing distinct models for "African sexuality," often obscured the moral and emotional aspects of African relationships, resulting in ahistorical and one-dimensional models for African masculinity and sexual desire.[16]

The ways we speak of and express emotion reveal not only culturally varied emotional practices but also the ways that these practices may change over time. Throughout the twentieth century, African discourses about love were potent ways for groups of people to mark generational and other distinctions.[17] According to anthropologists Holly Wardlow and Jennifer Hirsch, companionate marriage and personal intimacy have emerged as idealized representations of "modern" love across the globe.[18] They argue that the universality of such discourses about love (and the variable ways these ideals have been enacted globally) reflect the ways in which emotional registers are shaped by broader politicoeconomic and demographic shifts that make certain types of relationships more desirable and attainable than others. Romantic love has long been associated with the advent of economic change (in particular, the introduction of capitalism) that allowed for young people's economic independence from kin, thereby permitting the possibility of love unfettered by the larger economic concerns of extended family.[19] Romantic love has been described as an "affective individualism,"[20] emphasizing the way emotional expression is enmeshed in such broader historical shifts. In non-Western societies, the emergence of romantic love has been associated not only with the expansion of a market economy but also with the advent of a "development discourse" emphasizing such values as self-sufficiency, choice, and consumerism.[21] For young people, especially, discourses about and experiences of love become a primary way that changing social values are enacted, commented upon, and resisted.

In Uganda an ideal of romantic love has emerged over the past several decades alongside a higher incidence of informal domestic unions, lower rates of marriage, and higher levels of young women's education.[22] Recent economic shifts, which have heightened economic inequality and increased the prevalence of monetary forms of exchange, have provoked a new tension surrounding the individualist ideals, such as autonomy and independence, that underlie the experience of romantic love. Romantic love is now a more universal ideal in Uganda, viewed as modern and distinct from the traditional relationships of older generations, and also harder to attain, seemingly unstable in practice—and thus a concept frequently subjected to criticism. Gendered conflicts, whether they be instances of violence against women or more mundane legal conflicts over the rights of marriage (see the Marriage and Divorce Bill, discussed in chapter 2), may be linked to such structural shifts and may help enhance a critical view of romantic love.[23] Discussions of love also reveal the ways such tensions are gendered in particular ways. Pressures to pursue ideal models for masculine and feminine behavior have shaped youth attitudes about love and relationships and brought up complaints about the opposite gender's behavior.[24] Understanding how youth have defined and understood the experience of love and faithfulness gives us a better sense of how young adults navigate these changes and how they view certain relationships through varied associations with levels of economic, social, and epidemiological risk.

In the pages that follow I examine what intimate relationships were like in Kampala in the early years of the twenty-first century, the ideals that youth expressed about their potential partners, and the criticisms of nonideal ways of behaving and loving that arose. I then return to the Christian idea of faithfulness and the ways it emerged in contrast to these other models. Faithfulness was embraced by young people as an AIDS prevention strategy because it allowed them to critically reflect on the problems they associated with two other dominant models for "loving" relationships in Kampala: the traditional bonds of family and the pursuit of a secular romantic love. In particular, Ugandan youth employed the language of faithfulness to resolve the tensions surrounding forms of material and emotional affection that coexisted in both traditional familial love and romantic love. Love demanded money, youth complained, and this made such love "insincere."

The Provision of Modern Love: Money and Affection

On the Saturday nights when Makerere University was in session and students were on campus, youth leaders affiliated with UHC organized a free event near the university's outdoor pool that regularly drew hundreds of undergraduates. It was a raucous, happy event that many students looked forward to attending. The pool itself was an inspired choice for the weekly show, which was first staged in 2002 and has since become a student institution. Every week students clamored over the walls surrounding the pool grounds and spread out on the lawn at its edges, settling in for the evening's entertainment. It was certainly the most popular regularly scheduled form of student recreation on campus while I lived in Kampala. Yet it was distinguished from other events by its mission, which was to promote youth abstinence and planning for faithful marriage. The show was part rally, part concert, and part church service combining performances by visiting musicians with participatory games, skits, and—always included at the end—a sermon or lesson by a visiting pastor. The draw of free entertainment for cash-poor students certainly explains some of its popularity, but the organizers of the show claimed that their message was also an attraction for students who had become disillusioned with campus social life—especially romantic relationships.

One of the most popular recurring skits was a mock rendition of the nightly national newscast. Two announcers mimicked the familiar sonorous tones of the television anchors, reading the leading (fake) stories from around campus and Kampala. Reports often made fun of students' lifestyles. One story covered the "outbreak" of stomach cramps caused by overconsumption of the "rolex with beans," a cheap street food of fried chapati and stewed beans that was a staple of student diets. More often, however, stories returned to the themes of sexuality and relationships. Another report was titled "Condoms are in the ATMs." The actor, in his best stern newscaster voice, reported that "ATMs are now distributing condoms onto the streets of Kampala. This is making condoms ever available to the evil Ugandans who are prone to copying behaviors from abroad." He continued with the warning that "everyone who's been to school knows that condoms are not 100 percent safe, and in fact have a 17 percent failure rate."

Setting aside the actor's misguided lesson about the failure rate of condoms, the skit was humorous to students because it spoke to widely held beliefs about the state of sexual relationships on campus—especially the ways in which concerns about sex were inseparable from broader concerns about money and status. Men and women would share jokes that lambasted the traits of the opposite sex, and campus slang seemed to specialize in terms that pilloried perceived misbehavior in romantic relationships. Women were often accused of "detoothing"—extracting gifts and money from their lovers like an eager dentist with pliers. Men were "benchers," lazy hangers-on who would wait in women's bedrooms (on their benches) until the women finally acquiesced to sex. Attitudes about sexual relationships were often hard to separate from criticisms about overt materialism and an overemphasis on consumption in contemporary life. Both men and women felt that relationships were often extractive, where each party was being "played" by a lover of the opposite sex who wanted to get "something for nothing." A typical complaint from the male perspective was voiced by Allen, a twenty-two-year-old university student: "Some boys, they sleep with empty stomachs because they've spent all their money with girls. And those girls, when that boy is now bankrupt, that girl is going to find another one. But for you, you're staying with an empty stomach. Now, what's the use of that?" The average man was portrayed by women as heartless and untrustworthy, more interested in pursuing women as "conquests" than as "lovers." Catherine explained how women viewed relationships on campus: "The guys, most of them just want to use girls. And they might even make a bet to sleep with you: 'I dare you to sleep with her. And I will give you this amount of money.' So this guy comes and wants to convince you [to have sex], and after getting what he wants, he just dumps you there and leaves you there like that. That's what people think about campus relationships, mostly."

Women and men frequently spoke about a lack of trust in relationships and the sense that they were being "used" by partners who were in pursuit of something other than the emotional connection that was so valorized in the popular soap operas and pulp novels avidly consumed by Ugandan youth. This was a critique that was associated with the sense that the promise of modern, companionate relationships had failed to materialize for students. Dating and other forms of romance were often portrayed as more desirable forms of partnership, in large part because they were set in contrast to the supposedly loveless traditional relationships of one's parents.[25] Yet on campus (and throughout Kampala), popular discourse surrounding modern relationships frequently highlighted the problems associated with the pursuit of companionate love. Often these criticisms pointed out the ways that true love was supposedly corrupted by its entanglements with money.

The condoms in the ATMs story animated this sentiment: the pervasive feeling that sexual relationships were inseparable from the pursuit and acquisition of commodities, that romance had become less about true love and emotional connection and was instead driven by the pursuit of wealth and power. Sexual relationships that involved condom use—this story argued—were reserved for the especially criticized, extractive sex that had come to epitomize anxieties about the influence of money on relationships. The ATM in the story effectively highlighted these fears. ATMs themselves are used by a tiny portion of the Ugandan population—even less so in 2007, when this story was told, than today. They were novel machines that represented a form of wealth acquisition that could produce anxiety in Uganda. (One friend told me he liked to joke that ATM stood for "another terrible mistake.") ATMs were ambiguous symbols because they typified a form of impersonal accumulation that was associated with the problems of economic production in modern times. An ATM transaction was seen as a method of wealth extraction that was performed secretly, away from prying eyes, and anonymous even to the tellers inside the bank. It also represented a foreign, technological solution to money acquisition that was unfavorably contrasted with older forms of wealth and value in Ugandan society—wealth that, in contrast to the "fast money" of ATMs, emphasized interdependence, obligations to others, and investment in social relationships. With their effortless, anonymous ability to produce money, ATMs heightened awareness of the seeming abstraction of consumption from production, particularly at the global economic margins.[26] They were machines of *this era* of capital accumulation in Africa, an era when gaping inequalities, expanding opportunities for consumption, and "fast" sources of wealth drew intense scrutiny and moral rebuke.[27] In the fake news story, sex with a condom was thus associated with an ATM transaction: fast, secretive, extractive, and potentially immoral. It was the type of sexual relationship that students had learned to mock and lament, representative of a broader matrix of social conditions that left young adults feeling disempowered and unsatisfied. Such associations allowed abstinence advocates to quickly segue into a criticism of the condom's validity as a prevention tool itself: it was as failure-prone as the relationships youth found so "costly."

Students in the audience hooted and hollered in approval of this mock news story, jeering the depiction of an ATM that would eject condoms onto the city streets. The sketch's power lay in the ways it spoke to student complaints about the effects of a certain type of modern sex. Other newscast sketches returned to this familiar theme: modern life and material desires could lead one to behave immorally and irrationally. On another night, the newscast led with the story, "Tear gas in town is causing global warming, making kids dress revealingly," in which the government's use of force during a street protest generated a sense of not only environmental and social, but also moral, chaos.[28] Here the problems of contemporary youth sexuality were seen in the fashion choices of young women. (Men's sartorial choices rarely rated notice in Uganda.) Their miniskirts and other "revealing" clothing was another sign of the commodification of sex and of the moral upheaval that money (and state corruption) was believed to bring.

The underlying criticism in the Christian students' sketches was that money seemed intricately bound to urban romance, and that such modern relationships were thus immoral and unstable, driven by lust and greed rather than by "faithful" love. Their sketches were so effective because they played off the ways love and money were almost inextricably entangled in discussions of relationships and the experience of love in Kampala.[29] Yet the intersection of material support and emotional bonds are not always portrayed in such a negative light in Uganda. When I asked a group of women in their twenties who did not belong to UHC to describe an ideal partner, their comments highlighted the ways a male lover was expected to provide material support for a girlfriend or wife. One woman described the more mature expectations of lovers that came when one left secondary school:

> Secondary school love is based on writing love letters, sending cards, pocket money. But after secondary school I was looking for someone to take care of me, give me some money—of course, take me out. It feels good to have a gentleman take you out and give you some eats. At the universities in Uganda you have the sense that if you don't have a man to take care of you, you aren't beautiful. So I should get this kind of guy who would take care of me. It was a bit different than secondary school love. An ideal partner was [now] someone who would give you support.

In general, relationships—especially those outside the church—were considered more serious if the time and money spent to strengthen the bond between the woman and her suitor were greater. Affection was expressed often in material terms. Such attention made this woman feel good about herself, even beautiful. Male support through gift giving and the coverage of daily expenses (like the gifting of "air time" cards for a cell phone, or even a cell phone itself) were common parameters women used to assess the seriousness of a male suitor. A cell phone was a particularly popular gift for a lover because it was considered a tangible tool that could bring the couple closer together. A man who gave such a gift, for instance, would expect to be able to reach his girlfriend without a hassle.

When I interviewed a group of men, they were also clear about the ways they saw love and money as deeply bound to each other. One man described gift giving on emotionally intimate terms even as he derided the practice. He explained that when a woman "shares" her problems, a man's response is supposed to be to solve such problems with money: "The girl always starts telling someone's [her] problems. For what? Because she thinks that now you're sharing problems. So she comes and tells you, 'Yesterday, I lost my phone.' So you need to go and buy her another phone!" Even as he complained about a woman's behavior, this young man also described the complicated overlap between emotionally caring for and financially supporting a partner. Emotional intimacy was expressed in material terms, in ways that were frequently criticized but also accepted as normal, proper intimate behavior.

Another man, expressing a similar criticism of women's behavior, lamented that such expectations seemed to indicate a lack of "love" in Kampala. "You know," he said, "to a certain extent, I think, in Kampala I have come to believe that there is no longer any love. You find that they [women] are attacking you because you don't have money. If your pockets run bankrupt, that's the end of you." These common complaints about women's supposed greed speak to the complex place of money as a factor within intimate relationships. What does it mean to say that without money "there is no longer any love"? Does money indeed buy love?

In AIDS research, the interconnection between sexual relationships and money has driven a great deal of interest. Scholars struggle to define the ways in which money influences intimacy. The terms *transactional relationships, sex work,* and *sugar daddies* (as well as *sugar mommies*) have been coined to trace the variable models for relationships that are defined in some way by the exchange of material resources or cash but are not considered in local cultural contexts to be prostitution. While all of these terms reveal the complex way exchange can be a factor of intimacy, much of this research begins where Western folk concepts of love end: love is imagined as an emotional bond unsullied by money; material exchange and social status should be secondary to the bond that connects lovers. These models offer ways for (mostly Western) audiences to move past a strict dichotomy of love and money to understand relationships as existing on a sort of continuum more or less implicated by the influx of money into a relationship. In Uganda I found a far more complicated terrain where the emotional experience of love was not so much muddied by money as love and money were inextricably bound to each other in ways that were considered both positive and negative. That is, Ugandans did not necessarily see the "materiality" of love as a corrupting influence. And yet, as historical changes have altered the ways that love and material support intersect, Ugandans have become more vocal in their criticisms of some of the monetary demands of love.

The Materiality of Love: Historical Conjunctures

In Uganda the interconnections between love and material support have their roots in the ways intimate relationships were traditionally forged. Marriage for most Ugandan ethnic groups was historically marked by a bridewealth exchange. In societies where cattle had been an important form of wealth (in Uganda, especially in the northern and western parts of the country), the primary component of bridewealth consisted of a gift of some number of cattle to be negotiated between the bride's and groom's families. In other parts of the country, including Buganda, bridewealth consisted of several key cultural items (for example, a gourd filled with banana beer) as well as such agricultural staples as grains, fruits, vegetables, and small livestock that would be presented to the bride's family by the groom's family. Such gifts were not considered the outright exchange of goods for a woman (though the tension elicited by the appearance of such an exchange precipitated early Christian resistance to the ceremony, and still provokes disquiet among Westerners[30]); they were—and still are—viewed symbolically, as an exchange that unites and binds two families together, investing them both in the success of the marriage. A marriage united by bridewealth is thus considered more "respectable." (In Buganda it is said to bring *ekitiibwa*, or honor, to both a man and a woman.) Far from objectifying a woman, such exchanges "*exemplify* rather than *threaten* the distinctiveness of human self-worth," notes anthropologist Webb Keane.[31] Bridewealth exchanges amplify a person's social and moral connectedness to others and intensify one's social interdependence as a mark of status; this is believed to strengthen the union.

The practice of bridewealth also highlights the ways in which care and support can be expressed in tangible, often material ways. A relationship is solidified and made meaningful through a man's physical acts and material investments: the giving of bridewealth, the building of a home. Women's care and devotion were similarly expressed through palpable acts. For instance, to cook for one's husband continues to be the ultimate expression of wifely devotion and to neglect to do so, or to do so badly, is the ultimate failure. Ganda women's care for their husbands traditionally included washing their partner after sexual intercourse. Attention to the physical care of the husband's body demonstrated respect for one's husband and reflected ideals for gendered comportment within marriage. Such "caring" acts were expressions of love. We often think of love as an intangible emotional state. But as Fred Klaits has described in his study of Tswana emotional registers, love "is something people do as well as feel."[32] In precolonial Buganda, love was a feeling and sentiment, but also an act that worked to bond people to each other, and they were often people who inhabited two distinct yet interdependent social positions. Love did not happen in a vacuum; it was shaped by the actions of others. Love, and the acts of care, devotion, and provision that defined the sentiment, linked women to men, making them accountable to each other and their respective families.

In this sense, loving someone was to enact and reinforce a relationship of interdependence. As I noted in chapter 3, love was not only reserved for speaking about intimate relationships; it was also the way that Baganda spoke of their relationship to the *kabaka*, or king, and how they considered the deployment of political power. The historian Holly Hanson writes that the kabaka was understood to love his people when he provided land for their work, and their work was in turn a demonstration of their love for him.[33] Love was made visible by a variety of actions and ceremonial and material exchanges, both intimate and not; it was believed that these actions and exchanges reinforced relationships of mutual obligation and codes of moral interdependence.

Since at least the 1950s, both traditional bridewealth ceremonies and church weddings have been increasingly viewed as high-status achievements, and they are often postponed or delayed indefinitely.[34] This has been due in part to the increasingly high costs of bridewealth and to the changing expectations regarding men's readiness for marriage. As I noted in chapter 2, a bridewealth marriage in precolonial Buganda was the most significant marker of adulthood, the recognition by a man's elders that he was ready for his own household. When he demonstrated his readiness, elders would organize bridewealth for him and provide him with land on which he would build his family's home. Today a significant amount of personal wealth is needed to be considered marriageable. Urban men are expected to have finished their schooling, be established in a career, and have a salary that supports rent, the buying of furniture, and the maintenance of a household before they attempt to formally marry. In the wake of such changes, informal domestic unions have become more common, especially in urban areas where land is scarcer and the costs of living higher.[35]

As unions became further removed from models of precolonial marriage—where the ideal of physical care and provision, the setting up of a household, and the maintenance of a relationship of respect between a husband and wife took precedence—monetary forms of care became more prominent in how people began to think about love, devotion, and intimacy. A song recorded in the early 1980s by the Kenyan band Shirati Jazz, highlights the types of complaints about romance that had become commonplace by that time. In a comical repartee in the middle of the song, characters representing a man and his girlfriend discuss their differing expectations of their relationship: "Why is it that a man pays for love very expensively?" the man asks. "It almost started as a natural instinct, but I can almost see it now slide into some commercial concepts." His girlfriend replies, "Well, whatever you mean, I believe it is very natural" while demanding that his love be demonstrated by buying her a car. The song is meant to be funny, but the jokes the singers make play off of common (male) perceptions of women's behavior in romantic relationships.

As the normative path to adulthood has been delayed and transformed, new models for adult intimacy and heterosexual domesticity have proliferated. But these new models, while transforming generational and gendered relations, have added a sense of tension and disquiet surrounding intimate relationships. Marriage is no longer a "given"; men more often than not delay marrying for years until they feel they are well established in their careers. Women are widely perceived as having more freedom to choose, but also to manipulate, their male suitors. Young men lament the difficulties involved in marrying, and chafe against the oversight of elders who often still play a decisive role in the young men's ability to start their own households. Women complain of men's lack of commitment to marriage, the delay of which poses more serious moral risks for women than it does men.

As elsewhere, expressions of love in Kampala reflect the historical changes to households and families experienced over the last century. Monetary support has become a dominant way to mark devotion; it is viewed as an extension of older models of intimacy that were also, in part, material. But money is also ridiculed and blamed for the growing tension between women and men and for the many problems people perceive as being endemic to family life. Young men's loss of status in the present economic environment relative to their female peers is experienced on intimate terms, and complaints about such changes are expressed on moral terms: women "misbehave" when they are deemed to be "extracting" money from their lovers.

While earlier forms of exchange (namely, bridewealth) had instilled moral and social significance on a relationship in ways that outlined the interdependence of husband and wife and their moral obligations to each other and their kin, money introduced a different quality to intimacy. Money has the unique potential to both liberate and alienate."[36] Its use is associated with the advent of modern individualism, the depersonalization of exchange, and the value attributed to personal choice and freedom. But money also "wretches the personal value from things" and makes exchanges less socially meaningful and at times more unstable.[37] Ugandan attitudes about love reflect such tensions. The romantic love associated with monetary giving is idealized as a highly desirable signifier of a new type of relationship of companions bound by mutual attraction and a sense of shared intimacy and trust. Yet at the same time, romantic relationships that exist outside of marriage are considered weak bonds that are less morally sound and can be easily discarded for something better—in a word, interchangeable. These changes have proved more burdensome for certain sectors of the population more than others: youth and women bear the brunt of social complaints about romantic love. Young men, in particular, lament current conditions in which the older, normative path to manhood has been closed off but the newer one—oriented such as it is toward monetary giving—remains the purview of older, more established men.

Sincere Love and the Pursuit of Faithfulness

For many of these reasons, Christian youth at UHC were ambivalent about the redemptive possibilities of romantic love. One of their common complaints was that romantic love was unstable in practice. In speaking about their intimate relationships, young men and women expressed displeasure with the opposite sex and frequently spoke with me about a deep lack of trust in their lovers. Modern love presented a dilemma: it was often framed as a partnership of deep and meaningful attraction that survives the meddling of controlling elders.[38] In popular discourse this was how youth imagined loving relationships. In a youth seminar on AIDS prevention held in Mubende, a rural district to the west of Kampala, I asked the assembled young adults, most in their early twenties, how they knew when to stop abstaining and instead practice faithfulness. Somewhat surprisingly, the word *marriage* was not mentioned by anyone in the group, but the ideal of a loving relationship was. One young man said, "[You] should abstain until, in your heart, you find someone you know is the right one. And afterward you will trust this person." Many of these young people's comments pointed to the difficulties and costs associated with marrying. (They also highlighted a weakness in the message of faithfulness itself: how do youth know how to discern a faithful relationship from a nonfaithful one?) But the romantic language of their comments also spoke to the ways that such relationships were an ideal shared by many Ugandan youth who felt that love might better protect them from HIV and other problems. Loving partnerships were marked by the expression of mutual attraction, intimacy, and trust within a relationship. Shanti Parikh, who worked with young adults in an eastern Ugandan town, found a similar idealization of such partnerships, in which youth emphasized feelings of emotional intimacy, trust, and mutual affection.[39]

For many, however, the bond of mutual intimacy seemed fragile, too easily dissolved, and too open to betrayal. Romantic love's complicated intersection with practices of material support seemed to feed into young people's criticisms of the problems of contemporary social conditions. For women and men alike, love brought up fears of deception and betrayal by partners. Those beyond university age especially expressed somewhat hardened views of the redemptive and liberating potential of love relationships. These were the complaints evident in the skits and comedic performances I recounted earlier. Romantic love was portrayed as a weak love, driven by desire—for money, or for sex—rather than by sincere emotions.

Unlike the characters portrayed in their skits, moral Christian persons were considered to be those who knew how to channel their desires into appropriate emotional experiences—namely, the embrace of God's love. This was a lesson at the heart of the Christian abstinence and faithfulness message: true love could come only after a struggle to manage sinful lust. It was also central to the church's teachings about Christian personhood and moral community. During one graphic lesson the study leader, Gideon, smashed a watermelon and scooped out its red flesh in his hands. As he marched in front of the assembled group with the juice dripping off his fingers, he explained that young people's hearts were as hard as the watermelon's shell; one's inner feelings were only accessible through a relationship with God. Faithful love was a love grounded in the sincere, emotional, and affective experience of Christian belief and faith.

Webb Keane, in his study of Sumbanese Protestantism, has highlighted the importance of the concept of sincerity to the production of modern Christians.[40] He argues that sincerity, as a language ideology embraced by Protestants (for it is only through the "sincerity" of belief and prayer that one "becomes" saved), provides the subject with autonomy and authenticity as well as extrication from material and social "entanglements" that plague less-than-modern persons.[41] Keane argues that Protestantism emphasizes the moral value inherent in demonstrating control over one's inner thoughts and emotions. Similarly, at UHC, "sincere love" established a focus on individual agency (particularly in regard to the sublimation of desire and the avoidance of sinful relationships) and the internal transformation and continual self-renewal that was emphasized in born-again salvation. This process of inner-directed change was highlighted by church leaders to distinguish Christians from non-Christians. The interior emotional world of believing Christians was set against the problematic "emotionless" relationships of traditional Ugandans and secular modern people whose forms of intimacy Christians believed were predicated on, and plagued by, belief in the power of nonhuman and ungodly actors: fetishes, ritual exchanges, and witchcraft. Lessons taught by church leaders used the concept of sincere love to convey an argument about modern Christian personhood that was meant to enable church members to distinguish between appropriate and inappropriate relationships and thus to achieve "faithful" love.

Sincere love was believed to be true because it was supposedly abstracted from money and from social networks; it was derived from faith alone. Such a love had a theological basis: the remaking of the self as emotionally genuine through the help of God. Central to this experience of personhood was the idea of self-reform and improvement, an emphasis on an interior moral progression produced through the tension between human free will and the sinful nature of every human soul.[42] A person has the power to control his or her sinful desires, to cultivate a bond with God, but is also always tempted by such desires and will sometimes fail to resist them. This is a powerful message for people who are seeking the love of their partners and families; it is a promise that the companionate intimacy promised by the rhetoric of romantic love is within reach. Through belief in God, and through a better understanding of oneself and control over one's own emotional state, one could achieve a genuine bond with a Christian partner, a bond that existed outside the meddling control of elders or the material demands of contemporary urban society.

In order to achieve better self-knowledge, projects in church focused regularly on semipsychological self-assessments. Youth were taught to evaluate their "temperament" (e.g., melancholic, sanguine, phlegmatic, choleric) to assess their personalities' weaknesses and strengths and to learn how to better relate to others. Reflecting on the problems of past relationships—especially those of the family—was a common theme. Youth were taught to become more emotionally sincere and to think about the emotional insincerity of other (cultural) emotional registers.

Sincere love was a concept that was especially used to describe the problems of "traditional" forms of love. The emotional bonds of (non-Christian) family were considered extractive and calculating; traditional families were characterized as rife with tension. The individual needs of people were played against each other: husband against wife, sibling against sibling, parents against children. These problems were often attributed to a lack of love—between mother and father, parent and child. "Loving" versus "loveless" relationships were drawn along an axis distinguishing (modern) Christian relationships from traditional ones. Youth often spoke of the problems with "African" parents and marriages as ways of distinguishing their own, newly forged identities and relationships from those of an older, supposedly traditional generation. Edward expressed this sentiment when he spoke to me about parenthood and love in the church. "One thing in Africa is that our parents have not been very good," he said. "They have not learnt how to love their children. . . . But in church I have learnt how to be expressive about love. . . . And really think, what relationship do I want around? Church has really brought me up in that direction. There are so many friends of mine who really blame their parents."

Despite young people's criticisms of their parents' love, in practice the concept of sincere love functioned to establish a more ambivalent, less dismissive, stance toward non-Christian family life. In particular, faithful love seemed to be an attractive model for relationships because it emphasized youth autonomy and agency while also providing young men, in particular, with a pathway to older forms of cultural power and social status. Specifically, the church's model was appealing because it provided youth support in their pursuit of a formal marriage.

Faithful relationships were ideally begun in church and cultivated under the watchful eyes of pastors. Instead of dating, couples were taught that they should "court" each other. Courting consisted of spending time together, frequently in coeducational groups and often at church. Couples were supposed to develop a chaste intimacy and sense of trust in each other over a period of about two years, after which time the couple could consider marriage in consultation with their pastors. This courtship relationship was made public for purposes of—as one young man termed it—*accountability*. The use of this term differed in significant ways from the emphasis on personal accountability that I have highlighted in PEPFAR more broadly. At UHC the term *accountability* was used to emphasize the role of the group in holding individuals to their promises. The suitor was "accountable" in the sense that he must be "serious about this girl" and not lead her on without the intention of marriage. By announcing his intentions to court a young woman he was making his feelings public, and the community was expected to support the couple in their efforts to remain chaste while they prepared for an eventual marriage. Courtship was distinct from dating in that it generally did not involve the exchange of significant gifts or large monetary expenditures; the promise between a man and a woman ensured that the young man would not have to "compete" to demonstrate his affection. His intended was "beholden" to him and no other. The use of this anachronistic term was intentional, highlighting how Christian courtship stood outside the demands of a secular modern world that had often frustrated youth desires.

The ideal of faithful love must be understood alongside the larger significance of marriage for Ugandan youth. The church's promise of a courtship safe from the material demands of the secular world extended to the community's support of the wedding and marriage itself. Youth were provided with monetary and organizational support from church members that enabled them to plan their church weddings and receptions on tight budgets and with short time frames, even in the face of parental resistance. Youth were also provided with counseling and advice so that they could engage their parents in conversations about marriage and especially about bridewealth. I knew of no Ugandan youth who would forego a bridewealth ceremony despite the complications and contradictions it posed for Christians. Young people were encouraged to "negotiate expectations" with parents and encourage parents to "be realistic." They worked with their parents and in-laws to agree to smaller than normal bridewealth amounts, and many of them delayed paying bridewealth until later, sometimes years after the wedding itself.[43]

Unlike complaints about dating expenses, complaints about the costs of bridewealth were comparatively subdued. Within the church the practice of bridewealth was a common source of discussion, one that provoked criticism, but the youth also viewed such ceremonies as practically and culturally important. Eunice, a devout member of UHC, spoke with me about her preparations for marriage to a similarly devout, but poor, member of the church:

> We are thinking about marriage, but just by faith. He has just finished [his degree], he has not fully started working. And in my culture you need cows. With brideprice, they ask for twelve cows. And a good one is about 600,000 shillings. But I talked to Mom and she said maybe

he makes six cows, and we look for cheap ones at 400,000 shillings. That makes about 2.4 million shillings, which is still a lot for him. Someone gave him an acre of land and he planted cassava. And I was telling him today that he should shift from [staying at his pastor's] home and he should rent and slowly buy a few things like saucepans, plates, cups.

Here Eunice described how they had "faith" that he would be able to raise the money necessary for bridewealth (about US$1,150) and prepare a suitable home for her and their future family. While she was negotiating with her mother about the appropriate amount of bridewealth to demand from her partner, she still viewed such preparations as appropriate and her fiancé's ability to comply as a sign of his readiness for marriage. As is also true for non-Christian couples, participation in a bridewealth ceremony conveys a moral and social status on a couple that cannot easily be disregarded by young adults.

A faithful, Christian union not only provided youth at UHC access to an idealized form of "modern" love (the companionate marriage) but also allowed them to acquire a deeply important status in the traditional realm of extended kinship relationships. To be married remained an extremely significant social status for adults in Uganda. One woman, a successful engineer living abroad, told me that without a marriage she would never be considered a success by her family: "Myself, even if I work hard, to the day I die there will be people despising me. Nothing else will matter." A marriage supported by the church was particularly appealing to young people because it provided a new pathway through which to further their position in society according to older norms and hierarchies. Marriages were often opposed by elders not because it was undesirable that their children eventually marry but because in Kampala marriage was considered a status reserved for economically well-established men, usually those in their thirties and forties. By encouraging younger people to marry, the church provided them with the means to manage and transform the ways in which they interacted with elders and acquired social status.

Similarly, faithfulness provided these young people a new way of managing many of the concerns they expressed about relationships between men and women. For men there was the perception that dating relationships eroded male authority, allowing women to play one man off the other, to the women's financial and social advantage. These complaints reflected male dissatisfaction with their economic prospects in a city where unemployment was high and young men felt that the opportunities afforded an older generation had passed them by. For women there were similar complaints about the deceptive practices of the opposite sex, the ways men made empty promises and were not "serious" about love. For women and men alike, the ideal of "true love" was seemingly out of reach, clouded by the pressing concerns of a modern world that—like traditional relationships—had pitted men against women. Faithfulness provided youth with discursive and practical ways to manage their ambivalence about the constraints of traditional families as well as their dissatisfaction with certain aspects of modern life and relationships.

Conclusion: Faithfulness in Context

The message of faithfulness as an AIDS prevention strategy was remarkable on a number of levels, but none more so than its claim to appeal to a supposedly universal human emotion. In Uganda, models for love and intimacy were varied, and the social and economic pressures surrounding sexual relationships pressing. If nothing else, the message of faithfulness seemed a vague one in wider practice. My experience at the youth seminar in Mubende was striking for the clear sense it conveyed that the economic pressures surrounding sexual relationships, and the long delays before marriage, made faithfulness a nebulous ideal. Faithfulness also significantly differed from earlier Ugandan efforts that attempted to intervene in adult sexual relationships. In the 1980s and 1990s, the Ugandan government had encouraged people to reduce the number of concurrent sexual partners they had. As it has since been widely acknowledged, such changes in behavior critically reshaped the size of Ugandans' "sexual networks," reducing the overall risk of transmitting HIV.[44] But those behaviors were quite distinct from the ideal that would be commonly promoted in churches two decades later. Faithfulness demanded devotion to a single partner and was predicated on an ideal of companionate marriage that was but one, nondominant model for intimate partnerships in Uganda.

Young people's investment in the notion of love does little to alter the problems associated with the message of faithfulness as an AIDS prevention strategy. In much of Uganda, economic pressures can heavily influence decision making about sex. At another rural abstinence education seminar I attended, a Ugandan worker for a nongovernmental organization (NGO) shared with me the results of a survey his organization had made of young men in a neighboring trading center. The men were asked if they would knowingly enter into a sexual relationship with an older wealthy woman, a "sugar mommy," who would be capable of supporting her young lover, even if that woman was known to be HIV-positive. Two-thirds of the men responded that they would take that risk, regularly exposing themselves to possible HIV infection in return for the material comforts that such a woman could provide them. While this was an unpublished survey conducted by an NGO, the results—even if only anecdotal—are revealing. People must evaluate perceived HIV risk relative to other kinds of social and economic risks. For some Ugandans the promise of a stable financial future would outweigh the high potential for infection that would come from a long-term relationship with an HIV-positive person. Without altering the structural constraints that influence how people evaluate such risks, the project of advocating faithfulness will have its limits.

These constraints are difficult for many wealthier, foreign observers to contemplate. It is ordinary for a Ugandan child to drop out of school due to a lack of money to pay school fees. Even relatively well-off and educated parents may struggle to cover these costs, and their children may be out of school for several weeks, or an entire term, as their parents strive to raise the funds again. These and other everyday financial pressures alter how sexual relationships are considered, especially in a broader social context where sexual intimacy has long been associated with other forms of care and support. As I have discussed in this chapter, historical changes to these models of love have only enhanced the materiality of sex, making financial and sexual decisions even more deeply intertwined.

For Ugandan Christian youth the embrace of faithful love establishes marriage as a "solution" (to use Pastor Thomas Walusimbi's term) to many of the anxieties they express regarding gender relations and family life. But as a broader HIV prevention strategy it exposes the ways changing social and economic pressures reframe experiences of love, family, and sex and presents new challenges for disease prevention. The increasing prominence of a new Christian discourse of sexual morality may also be making other behaviors and habits—multiple concurrent partnerships, the use of condoms—not less socially prevalent, but less socially acceptable. In terms of condoms, this can create an increased stigma associated with their use, reducing compliance in situations where participants know disease risk may be high. In multiple concurrent partnerships this can hinder the possibility of open discussion, increasing risk to those involved. This presents real problems for disease prevention in a society in which far from all adults and youth attempt to embrace a born-again Christian ethos in their sexual partnerships.

In the minds of its American sponsors, and on the ground in Kampala's churches, the advocacy of faithfulness seemed to be a model of love well suited to the neoliberal era. This was a love driven by the autonomous choices of youth, its power derived from individual agency over one's emotional state. This was a "true" love, supposedly disentangled from material needs and desires, and a "modern" transnational sort of emotion belonging not to any cultural or historical context but to this era of empowerment and individual responsibility. In this chapter I have attempted to show the ways in which the advocacy of faithfulness was embedded in a history of love and intimacy in Uganda. Young Ugandans employed the discourse on faithfulness to engage their fears and criticisms of other sorts of intimate bonds, both familial and sexual. But at the same time, theirs was an orientation toward love that was shaped by those very social realities.

PART III

❖

In a Policy's Wake

6

FREEDOM AND THE ACCOUNTABLE SUBJECT

Uganda's Anti-Homosexuality Bill

The first phase of the President's Emergency Plan for AIDS Relief (PEPFAR) funded AIDS prevention and treatment initiatives for five years, from 2004 to 2009. In 2009, under President Barack Obama, funding for the program was renewed for a second phase, but several significant changes were made to the policy guidelines. Notably, abstinence and faithfulness programs were no longer earmarked for one-third of prevention funds. At University Hill Church (UHC) in Kampala, Uganda, this policy change was interpreted as signaling a broader disinterest on the part of the U.S. government in "moral" approaches to HIV prevention. Church leaders expressed dismay that abstinence seemed to no longer hold a privileged place in the eyes of either Ugandan politicians or American funders. But this did not dampen enthusiasm for social protest within the church; members of UHC remained active proponents for "sexual morality," though by 2010 their focus had shifted from AIDS prevention to a heightened concern with the practice of homosexuality in Kampala. At the end of the first decade of the new century, church members had become involved in an effort to pass new criminal sanctions on homosexuality in Uganda, and they spoke openly about the cultural illegitimacy of a discourse of human rights and sexual equality that was being forwarded in response to the growing antihomosexuality movement in Uganda.

I have described in previous chapters the ways that abstinence and faithfulness were embodied techniques with which youth navigated two distinct moral systems and managed a swiftly changing neoliberal terrain. The antihomosexuality movement proved to be a project less amenable to such negotiations; even more so than Christian AIDS prevention projects, the backlash against homosexuality calls attention to the tensions surrounding the promise of "accountability" as a solution to problems of governance. Of particular concern is the way rights-based discourses have been used to forge and outline the "accountable subject" in what Western nongovernmental organizations (NGOs) and governments view as broadly positive projects that benefit society. These projects face stiff opposition in Uganda, however. The rejection of homosexuality within the community I studied highlights the sense of failure that shadowed the neoliberal promises of self-help and self-empowerment and the enduring sense of tension between models for moral conduct and sexual personhood that coexisted in Uganda.

The advent of the AIDS epidemic heightened the visibility of sexuality as a topic of social advocacy and debate in Uganda as it did worldwide. Yet, in the process, sexuality itself emerged as a relatively new point of political intervention, an aspect of the self viewed as a distinct platform upon which individuals may make demands of the state and other authorities. The idea of "sexual rights"—in particular, advocacy for sexual minorities—has generated a significant degree of controversy and disquiet in Uganda in recent years. When I returned for a visit to UHC in 2010 the community was deeply enmeshed in an effort to support a new bill restricting homosexuality. "The Anti-Homosexuality Bill," introduced by a born-again Christian lawmaker in 2009, proposed new, draconian measures—including the death penalty—in an effort to further criminalize homosexuality in Uganda. These actions were widely scorned in the international media and by foreign leaders. President Obama called the bill "odious"; Secretary of State Hillary Clinton stated that "gay rights are human rights" and called on Ugandan president Yoweri Museveni to block the bill's passage. In the years following the bill's introduction (a version of it was briefly made law in 2014 before being annulled by Uganda's Constitutional Court on a procedural technicality) the governments of both Sweden and the United Kingdom introduced measures that would limit the amount of foreign aid to countries that attempted to legislate against homosexuality. But these rebukes seemed only to strengthen the sentiment among many Ugandans that such a law was necessary to protect a distinctly African way of life from the encroaching, and morally suspect, influences of Western culture and its attendant "freedoms."

In previous chapters I have explored how sexuality has emerged as a key element of new forms of African subjectivity and governance in the current era, and I have emphasized how global discourses about sexual behavior and health were made meaningful within local constructs of personhood, well-being, and moral obligation. My discussion of the controversy over homosexuality in this chapter illuminates some of the limits and tensions surrounding such projects—the ways a related international discourse about sexual rights was broadly rejected by the same community of religious Ugandans. I explore some of the reasons behind this rejection and what it may reveal about the potential for transnational projects seeking to advocate sexual and gender equality—especially in the realm of sexual health.

As I have noted throughout this book, sexuality in Uganda has long been a moral concern, a set of behaviors that marked one's interdependent relationships with and obligations to others. In this sense sexuality has always been an intensely important aspect of Ugandan personhood, but it has not been viewed as a part of the self distinct from other components of that personhood. Rather, it has long been considered integral and inseparable from the experience of kinship, reproduction, and gender identity. To the contrary, in Western countries—for at least the last century—one's sexuality has been considered a discrete object of moderation, control, and legislation; it has also more recently been recognized as an aspect of the self that is rights-bearing. The movement for marriage equality in the United States is one recent and obvious example of such a shift. Sexual identity, similar to gender identity and racial identity, has been made the basis for arguments that propose that variations in sexual identification do not preclude one from claiming the right to legally marry. Sexuality is viewed as a distinct platform upon which individuals may make appeals to the state and claim rights and privileges under the law.

The identity of the homosexual—a category of social persons defined by their sexual orientation—has had a relatively short, but socially transformative, history in the West. While sodomy had long been viewed as a socially transgressive act, it was only in the last decades of the nineteenth century that the desire to have same-sex relations was pathologized as a medical disorder. In so doing, the singular act of sodomy was transformed into the basis for a new sort of social distinction, an interior quality of the self that demarcated a defined social status. Michel Foucault emphasized the significance of such a shift when he wrote in his *History of Sexuality* that "the medical category of homosexuality was constituted [in 1870] . . . less by a type of sexual relations than by a certain quality of sexual sensibility. . . . Homosexuality appeared as one of the forms of sexuality when it was transposed from the practice of sodomy onto a kind of interior androgyny, a hermaphrodism of the soul. The sodomite had been a temporary aberration; the homosexual was now a species."[1] As Foucault argued throughout the *History of Sexuality*, it is the work of social prohibition that elicits and makes visible forms of social subjectivity. By pathologizing the interior state of same-sex desire, homosexuality emerged as a discrete and inalienable aspect of the person. And as same-sex encounters were marked as the basis for a nonnormative sexual *identity* rather than as singular *acts*, that sexual identity could also be claimed, acted upon, used for organization and, eventually, made the basis for a claim of equality and rights-based privileges.

The social category of homosexuality and the idea of sexual rights are also contingent on a somewhat longer history of Western sexuality and personhood—particularly the emergence of a right to privacy and the expanding significance of the ideals of personal freedom and sexual liberty. Western views of sex are shaped by the Enlightenment's conception of it as a private, personal matter; this was a shift enabled by changes in how Europeans considered the role of the individual conscience in governing moral conduct.[2] Arguments made in defense of gay rights today depend upon these transformative and fundamental changes in how Western societies consider social subjects and moral agency. Rights-based language itself dates to the philosophical and legal shifts in eighteenth-century Europe, to the emergence of a model of the "free" and morally autonomous individual.[3]

This is all to say that the critical response to Uganda's Anti-Homosexuality Bill has been forged on terms that have a distinct social history and depend on particularly European constructs of sexuality, personhood, and moral agency. Criticisms of the bill have by and large used the language of human rights—or, more specifically "sexual" and "homosexual" rights—to argue that the bill is unjust. I found that the rejection of homosexuality in Uganda seems to be linked to a disquiet about what this newly visible category of sexual rights means. Ugandan discourses surrounding homosexuality reveal a deep ambivalence over an emergent construction of sex and sexual desire that emphasizes individual autonomy, choice, and agency and conflicts with other models for ethical sexual conduct in Uganda. If abstinence was a practice that obscured and mediated disquiet over this emergent model of sexual personhood, homosexuality has uncovered and exacerbated it. It is this difference that interests me, and to which I will return.

My approach takes a critical departure from some of the most popular interpretations of the recent controversy in Uganda—especially those that have dominated Western media coverage. Much attention has focused on the personal connections between the sponsors of Uganda's bill and American religious conservatives. American Christian missionaries are believed to have counseled their Ugandan counterparts about how and why to engage homosexuality as a political and social issue, supposedly providing the impetus for this legislative effort.[4] I do not discount the significance of such connections, yet in analyzing this bill as simply the result of the transposition of an American homophobia we misrepresent Ugandan concerns as mere reflections of an American agenda and obscure the motivations of local activists. More significantly, such an interpretation fails to recognize the distinct moral conflicts and models of sexual subjectivity underlying American and Ugandan objections to same-sex relations.[5] Just as the subject position *homosexual* has a particular history, one that may be experienced differently in different societies, the meaning and force of homophobic discourse has also formed its own unique trajectories. American and Ugandan antihomosexuality activists may aspire to the same goal—the moral rebuke and criminalization of same-sex acts—but their motivations, and the underlying moral frameworks that shape them, are not interchangeable.

I am particularly interested in how arguments against homosexuality are imbued with a particular force and threat in Ugandan communities, especially given the ways other projects that seem to align with the ideals of personal freedom and self-empowerment—namely, the abstinence movement—have experienced relative success even in the very same religious communities that have so ardently protested homosexuality. The struggle over AIDS prevention and the conflict over gay rights highlight two interrelated aspects of contemporary forms of international governance and aid—the mutually constitutive ideals of accountability and personal freedom. Yet one of these concepts has been embraced by urban Ugandans, while the other has been scorned by a large sector of the population. Discussions about the meaning and effects of "freedom" are central to the ways Ugandan Christians speak about their rejections of rights-based claims to homosexual equality. Freedom is not viewed as a neutral value; it often emerges in discussions of homosexuality as a sinister, even dangerous principle, one that might undermine social values and ways of being that are seen as moral and worth preserving.

In the sections that follow I aim to show how the now infamous imagery that has emerged from this crisis over homosexuality—imagery that presents homosexuality as extractive, excessive, and perhaps spiritually dangerous—is emergent from and seeks to mediate the particular anxieties of the current era. Similar to the tensions underlying the message "abstain and be faithful" that I have described in earlier chapters, much of the anti-homosexuality rhetoric in Uganda is animated by a persistent conflict between two frameworks for ethical personhood: one related to the Ganda value of *ekitiibwa* (respect or honor), and the other based in a discourse of rights, autonomy, and freedom. But unlike the practice of abstinence and faithfulness, the discussion of homosexuality has heightened rather than alleviated the sense of moral conflict surrounding sexual behavior in Kampala. This tension elicits not only the rebuke of homosexuals but a palpable sense of spiritual anxiety and fear among many Ugandans. I describe how these fears are being generated in part by growing inequalities that have introduced new forms of instability that threaten to undermine the social hierarchies and experiences of gendered and intergenerational interdependence that have long defined Ugandan sociality and selfhood.

The Homosexual Controversy in Kampala's Born-Again Community

When I returned to Uganda in 2010 and 2011 it was difficult to miss the increase in popular interest in and discussion of homosexuality both within churches and on the streets of Kampala. Taxi touts and young *boda boda* (motorbike) drivers had made the bumper sticker slogans SAY NO 2 SODOMY; SAY YES 2 FAMILY and EBISIYAGA TUBIGOBE (We should drive out homosexuality) popular vehicle adornments (see figure 6.1). Street demonstrations in support of the African family were staged, and the topic of homosexuality and the

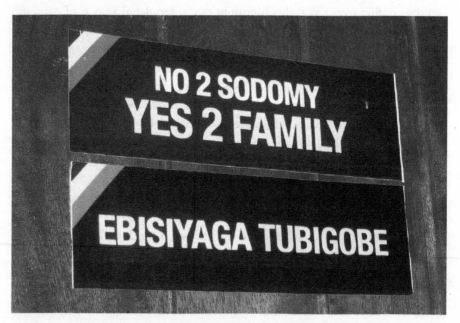

FIGURE 6.1. "We should drive out homosexuality"

Anti-Homosexuality Bill regularly made the daily newspapers. Members of UHC were also deeply involved in and affected by the controversy surrounding the bill. Pastor Walusimbi held demonstrations and press conferences in support of the bill and he had spoken alongside its legislative sponsor, David Bahati, to defend and promote it. The UHC youth group that organized weekly abstinence rallies had also worked to promote the bill after it was proposed in the Parliament of Uganda. Young people were encouraged to contact their parliamentary representatives, and the group considered different strategies for promoting media coverage and popular support for the bill, neatly recording their ideas in a binder that documented their history of activism and public engagement. This very public role as antihomosexuality activists had also made the church a focus of international criticism. During my most recent trip to Uganda, church members seemed fatigued by the strain of their efforts and the ensuing backlash. Church leaders spoke with me about their concerns in the wake of the withdrawal of donations from several American churches and Christian organizations, which they attributed to negative portrayals of Ugandan Christian support for the bill in the Western media. Because of this, members had also become more suspect about foreign interest in the church and were wary of any sign of unwanted attention. During my 2011 trip I arrived at church only to have a new member intercept me at the door and ask me to identify myself; the usher later explained that the screening of foreign visitors had become church policy.

There was a pervasive feeling that the sort of social activism that had once been so effective in garnering money and support from abroad suddenly had quite the opposite effect. This generated a sense of confusion and resentment, which often translated more broadly into criticism of Western motivations. As one member of another church explained to me, "When you come and talk about homosexuality, when there is a mother who can't feed her children, how does this make sense? Why does the West care more about homosexuals than those who suffered under the LRA [Lord's Resistance Army]? This is how it seems. This is what it seems human rights is."[6]

In many ways pastors are the ultimate "translators"—to use Sally Merry's term—who have sought to interpret, and in this case counter, the social significance of sexual rights-based discourses.[7] My focus here is on the ways pastors draw upon emergent tensions over models for moral personhood to help shape the debate over homosexuality within the broader Ugandan public sphere. In churches, homosexuality was placed in tension with the related discourse about sexual self-control—the management of one's body and desires—that was evident in pastors' advocacy of sexual abstinence before marriage. As much as abstinence seemed to mimic a neoliberal focus on the individual in projects of social transformation, I have discussed in previous chapters the ways it also reinforced older notions of ethical sexual subjectivity and behavior, an idea often simply referred to in Luganda as ekitiibwa or in English as "respectability." In many ways, the work churches did to promote abstinence sought to mediate between the seemingly opposed experiences of autonomy and interdependence and the ethical and cultural implications that both ideals carry. Homosexuality presented a new front in this struggle, especially as antihomosexuality sentiments articulated deep anxiety over a particular neoliberal construct of the sovereign, self-empowered individual. Below I examine how the idea of sexual freedom provided a counterpoint to "respectability" that animated social tensions concerning sexual behavior and shaped church leaders' arguments—and broader popular discourses—against homosexuality.

"Respectability" and Freedom: Moral Personhood and Sexuality in Buganda

In Uganda, attitudes about sex continue to be deeply shaped by notions of kinship and lineage that tightly bind experiences of sexuality and reproduction and, in turn, shape ideas about ideal gendered behaviors.[8] As I discussed in chapter 5, the most radical transformations to intimate relationships in the latter half of the twentieth century in Uganda and other parts of Africa may be marked by a growing emphasis on personal choice and mutual compatibility during courtship. Yet even as these changes have emphasized individual emotional and affective bonds, there endures the notion that one's identity and sense of self are deeply shaped by relationships to kin and by one's ability to reproduce.[9] In my interviews with young men and women, the interrelationship of marriage, reproduction, and the management of kin relationships was frequently emphasized. One young woman told me, by way of explaining the continuing importance of bridewealth exchange, "If he hasn't introduced [paid bridewealth], they will ask, 'Who is your husband? We don't know him. What has he brought here?' He won't be given any respect."

In contemporary Buganda and surrounding regions, respectability continues to delineate a way of behaving that reinforces relationships defined by reciprocal obligation and, in the realm of intimate relationships, is largely marked by the maintenance of kinship ties and the pursuit of formal marriage. Even today, a woman will still claim that marriage is the most significant social status she can achieve. One woman told me, "You are supposed to get married to gain respect." Another said, "However rich you are, if you don't have children no one respects you. If you are a woman, no one respects you without being married." This is not to say that men and women in contemporary Kampala do not have many sexual encounters that are driven purely by spontaneity, pleasure, and excitement. The Baganda are noteworthy in sub-Saharan African societies for claiming an erotic culture that exceeds a reading of sexuality as simply an extension of the functional power of kin and lineage.[10] And, as I noted chapter 5, since at least the late colonial era many Ugandans have engaged in long-term sexual and domestic partnerships that have not been formalized by a marriage recognized by kin. Yet the status bestowed through a marriage by bridewealth—even as other possibilities for domestic partnerships have emerged—speaks to the ways sexuality and reproduction are still embedded in a particular experience of kinship that is often expressed through the ideal of "respectability."

What has only occasionally surfaced in discussions about sexuality during this controversy has been the fact that same-sex acts have, of course, always been practiced in Uganda. I was surprised when Pastor Walusimbi owned up to this in an interview, especially given the way he and his peers have established themselves as guardians against this supposedly "foreign" practice. In his acknowledgment of the fact he clarified that it was not the mere presence of same-sex acts, but their acceptability for all—the universal "right" to homosexuality—that signaled a new, particular threat. He told me, "Sexual perversity has always been there. The difference now is that evil is not being combated. It is allowed to persist without resistance. . . . This attitude is new." The distinction he made highlights how same-sex acts have long been viewed in Uganda in terms of a freedom from cultural norms, the selective access to which marked social status or distinction. Kabaka Mwanga, who as a king of Buganda in the 1860s took liberties with many of his young male pages, is perhaps the most famous example of the ways a transgression of sexual norms could mark one's power and status.[11] Such distinctions are also evident in the ways homosexuality has long been viewed as an "imported" practice associated with a cultural "other"—not, at first, Westerners, but the earliest non-African "outsiders," Arab traders.[12] What is significant about these recognized instances of sexual "liberty" is that they were viewed in ways that reasserted relationships of hierarchy, status, and distinction. They emphasized the ultimate authority of the *kabaka* (king) or the cultural difference and superiority of the Ganda people themselves. These were not practices universally available but ones that, once claimed, marked and maintained social difference, dependence, or exclusion.[13]

This emphasis on status and interdependence contrasts with concerns about what other forms of "freedom" are thought to do in Ugandan society. In discussions about sexuality, freedom was often used to explain how problems arise when individuals became too independent—loosed from the constraints and expectations of kin. Young people were especially vulnerable to such criticisms—from within their own ranks as well as from their elders. A male student explained to me the ways in which a newfound sense of independence and freedom could be appealing but also dangerous: "There is a lot of temptation, and a lot of freedom [at the university]. We grew up in tight families and our schools are so tight. So, campus, it was like being released from bondage. And it was not just me; a lot of us got lost because it was like, 'Our freedom has come!' " Freedom was made to stand for a sort of loss of control, an inability to self-manage the myriad decisions and choices that marked contemporary—and especially urban—life. It was also used to mark non-Ugandan values and ways of acting, especially in the context of homosexuality, where a discourse of rights and equality defined opposition to the Anti-Homosexuality Bill. As one pastor chided his congregation from the pulpit, "Freedom has become an object of worship before God. That is how they can come here to tell us we are free to marry a cat. You shouldn't acquiesce to the demands of the West, to the allure of their freedoms!"

In Uganda, discussions about the "problems" of freedom seem to uncover an ethical tension over expectations for moral behavior in which older frameworks diverge from a liberal ideal of the sovereign social agent. These tensions are revealed in the contested definitions of what freedom means and how "rights" may be best actualized and managed. In Luganda, the term *human rights* is usually translated as *eddembe ly'obwebange* (personal rights) or *eddembe ly'obuntu* (rights of the people, or civil liberties), the latter also being a translation for *democracy*.[14] (The root, *eddembe*, carries the dual meaning of "liberty" and "peace.") As Mikael Karlström has argued in his essay on Ganda interpretations of democracy, this duality is important. The key point underlying his discussion is that within Ganda frameworks for describing the practice of democracy, the assertion of individual rights should always reinforce (and not oppose or threaten) established social relationships and hierarchies, ideal ("civil") relations between ruler and ruled.[15] Here it might also be significant to mention that, in Luganda, "human rights" is expressed in

IN A POLICY'S WAKE

the singular, as one "peace" or "liberty" of the people, a fact that may also reinforce this unifying, relational experience of rights.

This Ganda interpretation of rights emphasizes a distinct ethical framework based on the good of social interdependence rather than individual autonomy. Similarly, anxieties about the mismanagement of freedom reveal concerns about an erosion of ethical constraints that once shaped and channeled individual moral conduct. For instance, in terms of family and gender relations, unfettered freedom has often been viewed as a threat to the normative hierarchies that order society and social good. One young born-again Christian woman drew on this argument in response to my question about why homosexuality had so recently become a point of concern for Ugandans. "It is here now because of the changing society, the infiltration of Western culture," she told me. "There is too much freedom. There is children's rights, CPP [child protection policies]: don't cane at school. But we are still coming out of the African culture where a child is groomed. If you say don't cane, don't slap, and now that is made a rule, a law, now a child is free to do anything. So most of the infiltrations from the Western culture have caused too much freedom. If you don't control them, they do anything. They watch pornography." This young woman emphasized a perceived tension between "rights," which are viewed as mechanisms for independence from family discipline (thus eliciting the likelihood of misbehavior), and the moral cultivation inherent in the family's hierarchical relationships. Concerns about women's sexuality—often raised by male elders in an effort to control or manage it—have historically been expressed in similar terms, where migration and ensuing independence from male elders is thought to elicit—and, more generally, mark—morally suspect behavior.[16]

Freedom often came in the guise of the disordered, chaotic city, where immoral decisions were difficult to avoid. A story told by a member of a prayer group I attended highlighted the tension generated by the ethical management of new personal freedoms associated with urban life. Paul was from Teso, a region in eastern Uganda where daily life has been disrupted by Uganda's ongoing civil war with the LRA, causing waves of migration that have dispersed extended families. Paul told me that he had run into a friend who wanted to introduce him to his new girlfriend. Paul told them to meet him at his workplace in Kampala, where the three of them encountered another Teso man. This new man remarked that he knew Paul's friends and that they were both cousins of his (meaning they were themselves related, and thus forbidden to marry). All of them despaired and the couple lamented

Freedom and the Accountable Subject

their terrible luck. Paul recounted this story as a warning about the dangers of premarital sex and the necessity of a traditional marriage ceremony through which the extended families could formally affirm the identities of both the bride and groom. Fears about unintended incest—which were recounted to me in numerous similar "warning" stories by proabstinence advocates—reveal the ways moral transgressions are often associated with a breakdown of the authority vested in kin and lineage. As one becomes "more free," moving away from elders and engaging in sexual relationships in town without the knowledge of local clan and family leaders, youth are also more vulnerable to these sorts of (even unintended) morally and socially dangerous decisions.

Today's concerns about sexuality and freedom may also be especially shaped by the changing status of men and their relation to women. Unlike the colonial period, where men's authority and models of ideal masculinity were altered but also reaffirmed through institutions of the school and colonial bureaucracy, the present day posits far more unstable claims to male dominance. As I noted in chapter 5, pathways to modern manhood—through formal marriage and a wage earning job, for instance—have become more elusive, threatening young men's sense of their status and social roles.[17] Anti-homosexuality discourses reflect these tensions, especially as they manifest along an axis of intergenerational strife. The specter of an ominous, predatory older male sexuality—one that especially threatens young men—seems to have particularly dominated the current controversy. Older men are characterized as "recruiting" and preying upon vulnerable younger men, indoctrinating them into a "homosexual lifestyle." There is a related feeling that male desire has become unmoored, perhaps even dangerously unregulated and uncontrolled, in the contemporary era. These anxieties help inform the sense that traditional means of managing and channeling sexuality and desire in socially productive ways are eroding. As I will discuss below, this controversy has problematized male sexuality especially, revealing young men's growing frustrations with the neoliberal city.

Homosexual "Recruitment": NGOs, Intergenerational Tension, and Immoral Desire

Stories about the vulnerability of youth to homosexual advances have dominated arguments in defense of Uganda's Anti-Homosexuality Bill. In one of the most notorious public statements on the topic, a prominent Kampala pastor vividly described the physical trauma of anal sex, claiming a boy he counseled had died from the resulting wounds and that such youth were the hidden victims of the predatory tendencies of homosexual men.[18] Schools and churches, places where children are often separated from their parents and prone to the influence of other elders, have been characterized as likely sites for "recruiting" homosexuals.[19] In 2007 at a rally protesting homosexuality, Minister of Ethics Nsamba Buturo stated that no one "should be allowed to pursue an agenda of indoctrinating our children to homosexuality." The government, Buturo continued, was investigating reports that homosexuals had "infiltrated" schools and that some victims had died.[20] In 2008, government officials reiterated the fear that schools had become "breeding grounds for vice" when Minister of Education Namirembe Bitamazire announced an investigation into homosexuality in schools.[21] The 2009 Anti-Homosexuality Bill has been favorably compared by its supporters to Ugandan laws against child sexual abuse, statutory rape, and "aggravated defilement."[22] In a meeting with U.S. State Department officials in December 2009, David Bahati and a Kampala pastor attempted to defend the new bill from American criticism by forwarding the argument that the new legislation was an effort to protect minors from sexual exploitation.[23]

Among supporters of the bill, homosexual relationships are often described and critiqued through the idea of "recruitment,"[24] the perceived need for homosexuals to seek out and "initiate" others (usually children and young adults) in order to reproduce their way of life because they exist outside normative kin relations and are unable to have children of their own. This view reinforces the idea that sexuality is understood to be a function of other aspects of the self—especially gender and kinship roles. Many Ugandans expressed confusion over how homosexuals could "multiply" or regenerate without sexual reproduction. An example of such arguments about the nonnormative nature of homosexuality came from a Ugandan acquaintance who wrote in response to a Ugandan friend's Internet post, "I can tell [you] that in my region where I grew up, there are no homosexuals, and so I wonder where that habit comes from and becomes a normal sexual orientation. . . . How do homosexuals procreate?" His implication was meant to be quite sinister. If this was a sexuality that existed outside of kinship roles, where and how did people "learn" such behaviors? This argument was similarly put forth by another Ugandan on an Internet forum in response to an article about the bill: "As Ugandans, let us strongly come out to condemn this primitive and inhuman practice that the West wants to plant in our uprightly moral African society in the name of human rights. . . . The question I have always held is whether there [*sic*] are normal human beings??? Do they have parents, siblings, etc." The writer of this post above moves deftly between two related concerns: that homosexuals are operating in conjunction with Western norms and values that are threatening, even "inhuman," and that they are so dangerous (*not* "normal" humans) because they are supposedly unconnected to kin, clan, and lineage relationships.

A crucial element of Ugandan discourses about homosexuality relates to this anxiety. It is a sexuality to be feared not just because it marks a group of people as different but because the practice of homosexuals—seeming to reject reproduction outright by supposedly refusing or being unable to have sex with someone of the opposite gender—marks such persons as highly suspect, even antisocial. The disquiet generated by homosexuality seems to stem in part from the ways an assertion of sexual rights necessitates a decoupling of sexuality from kinship, gender, and reproduction. In response to my question about whether two men could marry, a woman I interviewed responded, "I don't count it as marriage, because who is a man and who is a woman? Who is catering [sexually] for whom?" When I continued by asking if marriage is "about sex" she answered, "Yes, it is the biggest thing . . . and how can they [two men] 'meet' [sexually]?" The mechanics of homosexual sex were not beyond the point for her; they were rather central to it: What kind of sex is this if these two men cannot reproduce? And what sorts of persons claim to engage only in a sex that can never be reproductive?[25] As one pastor explained in less generous language, "In America homos have rights. Here you have no rights. You are not even a person. You are outside society because you are not acting like a person." Asserting equal rights to sexual behavior that is seen as challenging other elements of moral personhood—the ability to reproduce, for instance—is disconcerting for many Ugandans and, in the context of debates over this bill, made to seem deeply threatening.

A key element of homosexual "recruitment" stories builds on these fears by associating homosexuality with foreign money and power that may challenge children's allegiance to their families and elders.[26] The homosexual "recruiter" has emerged as a corollary to the licentious figure of the "sugar daddy," who has long animated anxieties about the vulnerability of young women to the sexual advances of older men in the age of AIDS. Similarly, the homosexual recruiter preys upon young people's economic vulnerabilities to lure them away from the safe and moral confines of their family. In one interview a man explained the sorts of tensions he believed existed between one's obligations to kin and the desire for money that he presumes most homosexuals must be drawn to. "In our clan, there are very few people who will like that [you are gay]," he said. "Because if they hear you are gay, very few will take a girl from your family. It is increasing because people are very poor. If they [homosexuals] come and say, 'I'll give you two hundred shillings,'[27] you will do it [have sex]. Then they will tell you to convince others. And you will. 'Why don't you forget about women! They are head-aches.' But if you go back home they will keep you away because you are an animal; you can do anything." Other men present during this interview interjected to explain that homosexuality, like leprosy or epilepsy, is con-sidered by them to be an illness that affects the clan's well-being and that must be treated by appealing to ancestral spirits. Because of this, when homo-sexuality is "brought home" it may inhibit the ability of everyone to marry properly. Here homosexuality is emphasized as a problem that exceeds the individual: beyond simply bringing shame to one's family, a homosexual is viewed as undermining other social relationships and obligations. (It might also be noted that homosexuality is interpreted as being appealing because it provides a way of gaining illicit monetary wealth while also circumventing the demands of female partners, who are widely accused by young men as levying heavy financial burdens on them.) In such stories homosexuality is constructed as a corrosive influence (in many ways, like other sources of ex-cessive wealth that is not equitably shared) that is the basis for new, immoral social ties that threaten older, normative ones.[28]

In March of 2009, several months before the new bill was presented in the parliament, a local pastor called a series of press conferences featuring the testimony of young men who spoke about their prior participation as "recruiters" of children. In their testimony, homosexuals were described as luring children—in these instances with consumer goods and travel—and "initiating" them into an elaborate organization funded by anonymous for-eign sources. In one Ugandan newspaper account of the event, George Oundo describes such techniques: "'I was taken to Nairobi for training,' he said. 'I used to supply pornographic materials in form of books and compact discs showing homosexuality to young boys in many schools,' he explained. The training, he said, was facilitated by [the] Gay and Lesbian Coalition. 'I also got the pupils' telephone contacts. We used to meet with both girls and boys in schools during ceremonial parties,' he asserted."[29]

Travel across national borders, ominous foreign "coalitions," and the sup-posed use of technology to recruit and train youth all play on fears about dangerous external forces that may gain influence over children. Money and mobility are especially potent signifiers that oppose and may undermine local forms of authority and social reproduction. By placing children at the center of discussions about homosexuality and depicting them as victims easily drawn to a "foreign" way of life, pastors and others deftly link homosexuality to other contemporary anxieties about social forces that threaten hegemonic relationships and social hierarchies. Such stories also highlight a deep anxiety about social reproduction during a period of expanding urbanization and capitalist consumption.

The deceptive lure and power of the NGO has especially dominated Ugandan "origin" stories that seek to explain the mechanisms and success of homosexual "recruitment." In the following story, told to me by a young man, the NGO is described as an entity that imports, finances, and organizes homosexuals:

> I know of an institution somewhere in Ntinda, just around the [taxi] stage. They opened up a house, and turned it into an NGO. And the prominent girl of a prominent minister runs that place. And they do that exercise [sex] in there, that place. And they get paid money. Actually one of the boys I grew up with here also does the homosexual activity there. . . . [My friend] goes to work at weird hours. During the day he sleeps at home and then he is having very many phones and he receives lots of calls. And he says, "Have you received the cargo?" And so I went to see them deliver the cargo, and they are getting shipments of flesh! Human beings! And then they take them to this place and they get paid a certain amount. Then they go and hang out in airports, shopping malls, supermarkets.

Here, as in other testimony above, homosexuality is linked to urban spaces associated with travel and consumption, desirable but also potentially dangerous places linked to a capitalist power that is viewed by many Ugandans as morally ambiguous. In this story, homosexuality is first and foremost a *job,* one that is deviant (working at night!) and driven by technology. It is also extractive and deeply immoral (buying and consuming "flesh").

Like other rumors in Uganda and elsewhere, the attempt to describe the source and terrifying effects of disordered power (in this case, the potentially extractive power of NGOs), these stories use fantastic elements to refract reality, addressing social anxieties relating to economic and social conditions.[30] NGOs take up a somewhat mysterious place in the popular imagination in

Uganda; they have what seems to be unlimited access to foreign money and support—a job at an NGO has eclipsed government work as the sine qua non of employment status—but their allegiances to local norms and hierarchies are often vague, especially in those NGOs that advocate rights-based challenges to promote the status of women and youth. This simmering dissatisfaction that links NGOs to "immoral" behavior and other social ills may also speak to changing experiences of governance in the neoliberal era, where the retreat of the state has been replaced by empty promises of individual freedoms and entrepreneurial wealth.

It should be noted that the predatory character that has dominated so many cautionary tales about homosexuality during this controversy has often highlighted a male homosexuality rather than a female one. Rebukes of lesbians in Uganda and other parts of Africa have been analyzed for the ways such backlashes seek to control women, to reassert normative gender roles and subservience to male authority.[31] The image of the predatory male homosexual seems also to relate to dissatisfaction with changing gender relations in Kampala and young men's anxieties and frustrations in their inability to dominate their relationships with women and others. But in this sense these stories seem also to take up a much broader critique of elder men's responsibility to, and perhaps abuse of, younger men; of the extractive and predatory nature of economic opportunity in contemporary Kampala; and of the marginalization and frustration that many youth, and especially young men, regularly express. Antihomosexuality sentiment may then be more than simply a reassertion of the authority of gendered and generational hierarchies in the face of social change. Such sentiments seem also to express a critique of traditional social norms that have failed to protect and provide for young men.

Secrecy and Spiritual Danger

I have discussed how homosexuality is constructed as a subject position set in contrast to the Ganda ideal of "respectable" persons that is based on the maintenance of normative kin relationships. I have also described how this description of homosexuality is animated by fears about social changes—especially those concerning the waning authority of elders over youth and the corrosive effects of certain types of wealth and power. But it is also important to understand the spiritual threat that such discourses produce, especially as such threats have come to dominate local interpretations of homosexuality in Kampala.

In Uganda, homosexual sex, like all sex, is thought to have spiritual consequences, for oneself and for others to whom one is related. As I noted in chapter 4, Ugandan born-again Christians often participate in intense deliverance prayer sessions, seeking to "cast out" relationships that are viewed as spiritually dangerous. Sexual relationships, particularly those viewed as illicit (for example, one of premarital sex), are believed to generate long-standing spiritual repercussions that must be addressed, usually through intense prayer that breaks the "soul ties" generated by the intimate exchange involved in such partnerships. The close scrutiny of relationships is a central part of spiritual work, where those ties that are socially and morally productive are separated from those that must be revealed, confessed, and then abandoned.

In the rhetoric of pastors, the danger of homosexuality has been especially marked by its relationship to acts of deception and secrecy, the willful obfuscation of nonnormative sexuality. Pastors often spoke about the need to reveal the illicit activities of homosexuals. The Anti-Homosexuality Bill's authors actually claimed that one of their goals was to "define" homosexuality, to delineate and expose practices that were believed to have been dangerously hidden from society.[32] In the now infamous press conference staged by the Ugandan pastor Martin Ssempa (and circulating on YouTube) the clergyman presents the results of "a little research" he undertook "to know what homosexuals do in the privacy of their bedroom." What follows is a graphic description and then partial screening of an American gay pornographic film featuring defecation. During his presentation—to an audience of Ugandan Christians, local media, and several visiting American youth missionaries—gay sex is portrayed as secretive, insatiable, and dangerously uncontrolled. By "disclosing" these hidden acts Ssempa seeks to mark them as especially problematic and antisocial.

To share a secret binds those who know from others who do not, a parceling and limiting of knowledge that establishes difference and authority. Secrecy, as Georg Simmel has argued, is central to the production of social distinctions and hierarchies.[33] In a similar sense, the revelation of that which is hidden carries special power to define and demarcate what is "other." In Uganda the revelation of the unspoken, the demarcation of an act as one that is and should remain hidden, may also mark that act as part of a spiritually dangerous "outside." Achille Mbembe remarks that the secret in African societies holds special weight: "the great epistemological—and therefore social—break was not between what was seen and what was read, but between what was seen (*the visible*) and what was not seen (*the occult*), between what was heard, spoken, and memorized and what was concealed (*the secret*)."[34] In this sense, the emphasis on exposure that has been evident throughout the recent controversy—perhaps most notably in the front page tabloid exposés that sought to name and "out" Ugandan homosexuals—becomes more than a public humiliation (or, more ominously, a call for violence and persecution). Presentations like Ssempa's seek to delineate and reveal, to mark homosexual sex as part of a spiritually dangerous "outside" to socially productive relations.

These acts also become a mirror for male sexuality more broadly: the abhorrent antithesis, the result of desires unchecked. "Disordered" images of defecation and sex in Africa (and elsewhere) are not, of course, limited to the representation of homosexuality;[35] such images tend to highlight dysfunctional social relations, the corruption of moral obligation and affinity between dependent social groups. Homosexuality, like incest (another dominant theme in morality tales in Africa), presents a particular disquiet in its disordered familiarity, its transgressive reversal of what is intimately known. Julia Kristeva's notion of the abject articulates how such images become effective. "It is thus not lack of cleanliness or health that causes abjection but what disturbs identity, system, order," she writes. "What does not respect borders, positions, rules. The in-between, the ambiguous, the composite."[36] In the images put forth by Pastor Ssempa and others, homosexuality is presented as something to be feared because it dissembles; it feigns normativity but reveals itself as its reverse, nonproductive other. Such images play upon the ambiguity and intensity of kinship relations and the inherent tension that proximity and dependence may elicit. A secretive, nonnormative sexuality, one that operates outside the bounds of relationships of kin and lineage that are thought to productively manage and control personal desires, is especially dangerous.

Such orientations reflect a cultural framework that views certain sexual misbehavior through the lens of the occult. In interviews, school dormitories often surfaced as places where girls especially were vulnerable to occult forces that would take the form of lesbian "spirits." One young woman explained that student prayer sessions in her school usually revolved around the shared interpretation of dreams of "revelation." "Being a girls' school, we would have cases of lesbianism," she added. Whenever people dreamt, the interpretation was either that the person was [possessed by] a lesbian or a devil's agent." The interchangeability between the figure of the lesbian and the "devil's agent" speaks to the ways homosexuality (perhaps especially lesbianism) is seen as a threat to the webs of interdependent spiritual and social relationships that underlie normative kinship ties. The connection between homosexuality and the occult may also be informed by the fact that witchcraft is often characterized as having a disregard for sexual norms, especially in acts that manipulate or transgress social hierarchies. In Buganda, for instance, *basezi* (night dancers) are witches who are believed to roam freely after dark, engaging in a wide array of mischief, and are identified especially by their antisocial sexual practices. They eschew norms of dress and behavior, dancing naked, entering compounds to rub their oversized buttocks against terrified neighbors' doors. Illicit sexual acts, especially those driven by the pursuit of money and at the expense of normative relationships, hold a special place in the popular imagination. In the Ghanaian and Nigerian films popular with many Ugandans, modern life is often presented as a morally fraught terrain, rife with unregulated sexual desires that are usually satiated through the occult pursuit of wealth and power.[37] When pastors and others describe homosexuality as a hidden, excessive, unreproductive type of sex unregulated by and in opposition to normative kin relationships, unmistakable parallels are drawn to other forms of dangerous, antisocial misbehavior—especially witchcraft.

This discourse plays upon fears about the changing nature of gendered and intergenerational dependence and draws upon a spiritual framework that views the seeming manipulation of such ties as socially and morally dangerous. If homosexuality is placed in tension with a traditional ideal predicated on the maintenance of kin relationships (and, in turn, "respectable" personhood), it is also used to express concern about the emergence of a new form of ethical subjecthood, one predicated on the embrace of personal rights and freedoms.

Conclusion: Neoliberalism and Human Rights

Many Ugandans I spoke with expressed the idea that certain rights could be antisocial, a means by which individuals might erode or directly challenge accepted modes of authority and standards of conduct in society. At the core of this conflict over human rights lie divergent models of moral personhood: one predicated on interdependence and obligation, the other on the neoliberal ideals of autonomy and self-empowerment. As Talal Asad has noted, we must "analyze human rights law as a mode of converting and regulating people, making them at once freer and more governable."[38] Asad and others have pointed out that human rights, particularly in the postwar era, when it became a widespread platform for social activism and political reform, is as much about shaping and governing individual conduct—the making of particular models of "liberal" persons—as it is concerned with bestowing freedoms and protecting equality.[39] In separate analyses, Harri Englund and Talal Asad have pointed to the shortcomings of rights-based discourse, and especially to the ways it may limit or obscure other frameworks for social action and organizing already present in diverse societies. In the case of Uganda such shortcomings seem to have played into a critique that characterizes such projects as especially foreign, threatening, and "un-African."

Throughout this book my discussion of conflicts over sexual behavior has been shaped by the idea that ethics is animated by more than a Kantian emphasis on autonomous, rational choice, or a Durkheimian reading of the moral code as a "total social fact." As James Laidlaw has argued, an anthropology of ethics is based in a recognition that ethics is about the making of a certain type of self: the choices, constrained by variable forms of social power, that shape individual efforts to create themselves in particular models of moral persons.[40] In Buganda the pursuit of "respectability," a value predicated on proper relatedness, emphasizes a model of personhood articulated through the proper reproduction of lineage and clan. Antihomosexuality activists have succeeded in constructing the homosexual person as an imminent threat to such ways of being and posing a serious moral danger to other persons and society. This is not to say that human rights inherently have no value in Ugandan society; nor do I mean to argue that "traditional" personhood and sexual behavior is imbued with an immutable authority in the lives of Ugandans. What I have illuminated in this chapter is how and why particular homophobic discourses have been made meaningful in the historical and cultural milieu of contemporary Kampala.

The homophobia that has reared its head in Uganda, just like the subject position of "homosexual" itself, is a historically contingent one. It has emerged within the context of neoliberal social conditions that have exacerbated social inequalities even as such policies have espoused the (elusive) power of the individual to change these conditions. Criticisms of gay rights are deeply intertwined in growing dissatisfaction about political and economic conditions, a criticism that seems especially directed outward to the realm of international organizations that shape local experiences (and failures) with "development." For at least some Ugandans, a privileging of the rights-bearing subject seems to pose a threat to other constructs of persons and relationships that are deemed moral; it is a threat that would appear to be evidenced by

Freedom and the Accountable Subject

the apparent disintegration of sociality in the context of an overcrowded, economically disenfranchised Kampala. While the political repercussions of such a discourse have not been the focus of this chapter, they should not be overlooked. President Museveni has weathered increasing criticism in recent years for what many see as his abuses of power deployed in an effort to maintain his control of government. The controversy over Uganda's Anti-Homosexuality Bill has served to deflect critical eyes—including those belonging to masses of dissatisfied youth and powerful members of the conservative elite—away from an examination of the Museveni administration's tenure and to focus criticism instead on an already socially marginalized and vulnerable group of people or, better still, the meddling interventions of Western diplomats and activists.

And yet, a discourse of human rights has not been without some success in Uganda. One need look no further than Karlström's discussion of democracy to understand how a seemingly foreign liberal value was reinterpreted in ways that was significant within local moral frameworks.[41] The women's rights movement has had a similar success, incrementally shifting the outlines of what "proper" womanhood entails, even if this has not as of yet engendered the wholesale embrace of gender equality in Uganda.[42] Homosexuality seems to pose a particular challenge for the reasons I have outlined here. But what these examples reveal is that efforts to advocate for sexual equality may be most successful by aligning with existing Ugandan frameworks for justice, dignity, and respect, and in the process shifting the outlines of what an ethical sexuality entails. What is painful to acknowledge is that current efforts have done little to counter what seems to be a rising tide of hatred and violence against gay people in Uganda. One need look no further than the 2011 murder of David Kato, a Ugandan advocate for gay rights, to realize that a successful counterdiscourse about homosexuality has still failed to gain any traction. Developing a meaningful connection to local notions of humanity may be a starting point. Perhaps most critically, such a discourse needs to be viewed as emergent from—rather than in opposition to—indigenous frameworks for moral action. As such, the outlines of moral personhood, and the contemporary meanings attributed to Ganda "tradition," may be reinforced in ways that encourage change and an embrace of sexual diversity.

In the born-again Christian community I studied, homosexuality became a cause that seemed to reflect and embody the problems with transnational alliances and religious ties between the Global North and the Global South.

As prominent evangelical Americans spoke out against Uganda's bill, those at UHC expressed frustration over the perception in the West, even among Western Christians, that their work advocating against homosexuality was without merit—or, worse, that its was un-Christian. More so than work on AIDS prevention, homosexuality was a cause that seemed to highlight rather than obscure the differences between Ugandan and American Christians. These were differences in resources that were emphasized when many of UHC's small-scale American funders withdrew their donations in protest in the wake of the negative publicity over the bill, but these were also differences in orientations to sexuality, moral behavior, and social action. The controversy surrounding the Anti-Homosexuality Bill revealed more than an emergent homophobia in Uganda; it was a conflict that highlighted the very different experiences of sexual personhood and moral action that shaped homophobic discourse and influenced Ugandan responses to the bill. These were differences that were integral to AIDS activism but were less obvious when the lens was focused only on the seemingly bilateral embrace of "abstinence and faithfulness."

EPILOGUE
Beyond the Accountable Subject

The research for this book was conducted within a community of Ugandan born-again Christians who were directly involved in advocating for and promoting the HIV prevention guidelines that were then being advanced by the U.S. government. University Hill Church (UHC) was a church that in many ways seemed far removed from U.S. policy making and religious politics. It was run by and served Ugandans. Yet it was also a place where faith, "development," global health policy, and American and Ugandan politics converged, where ideas about health and behavior were both promoted and contested. In that I have taken up the topic of an international policy's implementation in Uganda, this book has addressed how AIDS and epidemics more generally are never experienced as bounded, localized crises. Rather, policies such as the U.S. President's Emergency Plan for AIDS Relief (PEPFAR) are vehicles that conceptualize disease across boundaries, shaping and reconfiguring how health, risk, and blame are understood within particular communities.[1]

Much like other international development programs, global health initiatives such as PEPFAR mostly originate in the West and are oriented toward particular notions of what constitutes political engagement, economic "empowerment," and good health. As I noted in chapter 1, the current environment surrounding international development is in part shaped by the terms of neoliberal economic policies that have, for the last twenty years or more, cultivated certain values and forms of politics in recipient nations. These economic terms have established powerful new modes of governance through which individual choice, personal empowerment, and accountability have become the dominant forms of both political and economic engagement. I have argued that indigenous conceptions of political agency, moral obligation, and personhood have been largely sidelined by such broader processes in favor of a targeted focus on the cultivation of the individual rights-bearing and accountable subject.

In terms of health care such policies have focused particular attention on the regulation of the body and physical behavior. In Uganda the demonstration of physical need and the cultivation of personal improvement and "will" have become ever more important platforms upon which individuals may seek aid and upon which they are taught to become more "responsible" healthy citizens. PEPFAR's message that Ugandans should adopt behavior change strategies—that they should practice abstinence and faithfulness—was a lesson animated by these larger changes to the structure of aid and global health. Practicing faithfulness was not simply a reiteration of "traditional" values— even though members of the administration of President George W. Bush and Ugandan politicians and pastors may have characterized it as such. Being faithful became a way of thinking of oneself as "empowered," autonomous, and responsible. It was a new, distinctive way of being in the world and enacting morality. It was an aspirational message, and as such it was a way of behaving that was different from other models for ethical behavior that existed alongside it.

From the perspective of the American government and most Western observers, it is hard to envision the problems that a focus on personal accountability might have, especially when that accountability is understood to be animated by certain values that Americans hold dear, and especially as such values are associated with ostensibly morally unassailable projects like disease prevention and human rights. But projects shaped by the ideal of personal accountability were at once desirable and problematic for Ugandan youth, and the contradictions that these youth faced in adopting these strategies revealed the strategies' limitations as approaches to disease prevention. In part, the failure of the message of accountability was that it overlooked, and even obscured, Ugandan orientations toward sexuality and health.

The language of youth autonomy, of the power of self-control and personal empowerment, was deeply appealing to young Ugandans. But these ways of thinking about the social person were constantly challenged by spiritual and social frameworks that emphasized young people's obligations to the kin group and community. These conflicts went beyond the demands of family and the concerns of parents that young people respect "tradition"; they were conflicts about how people imagined health, proper behavior, and moral obligation. These moral orientations affected the ways that health was pursued, and they had an influence on Ugandan responses to messages of abstinence and faithfulness.

In many ways the embrace of abstinence by youth at UHC concealed many of the problems associated with the broader emphasis on accountable subjects within international aid programs. During the Bush administration, when religion seemed to emerge as a new, potent strand in international aid—one not tangential to American government aid programs but very much at the center of them—abstinence seemed to align Ugandan and American orientations to sexual behavior rather than highlight their underlying differences. For both Bush administration officials and Ugandan politicians and pastors, accountability was hinged to a broadly Protestant discourse about personal transformation through faith. In practice, however, young Ugandan born-again Christians struggled to navigate differing models for moral subjecthood. To be empowered and autonomous was a deeply desirable goal, but it had to be pursued in an environment where well-being had long been considered a collective pursuit, where one's health and prosperity reflected not an interior state of salvation but the ability to properly manage one's spiritual and social ties with others. The demonstration of interdependence—contributing to relationships of ongoing mutual support and obligation within one's kin and social group—continues to be more socially and morally significant to Ugandans than cultivating one's independence and self-reliance. As I have described in this book, youth used abstinence to navigate and contest these contrasting models for personhood and to make sense of an urban landscape of sexuality and family life that often left them feeling marginalized and disempowered.

When I left Kampala after my initial period of fieldwork in 2007, abstinence seemed to be a strategy firmly in favor with Christians and in the highest reaches of the government and development sector in Uganda. It was the theme of youth rallies in central Kampala, and it was spoken about at AIDS conferences held in the city's sprawling upscale hotels. At UHC, young people seemed energized by the sense that they were, as Pastor Walusimbi liked to remind them, "global leaders" in the effort to abstain. Uganda was widely recognized in the West for its apparent success with what was now known as behavior change.

When I returned to Kampala in 2010, the ground had seemed to shift, if subtly. A new American president had been elected, and the Ugandans I knew were keenly aware that he was not known for advocating the same sorts of social policies as his predecessor. The community at UHC was struggling to grasp the changing terrain of AIDS prevention and the international concern with sexuality and human rights that had formed in the wake of Uganda's Anti-Homosexuality Bill. Pastor Walusimbi voiced frustration with changes in funding patterns that had shifted resources away from abstinence-only education; he told me he believed that international funders were now dominated by what he called the "freedom-of" people, by which he meant people who used the language of rights and equality—rather than such concepts as tradition and self-control—to address problems like HIV/AIDS. He complained bitterly to me, "Freedom of—that whole description of, 'I'd rather have freedom than life. I'd rather die of HIV/AIDS than you tell me to exercise self-restraint.' Those guys have taken over."

Walusimbi's angry dismissal of the idea of freedom, a concept I discussed at length in chapter 6, highlights the fault lines that existed beneath the embrace of accountability as a mode of moral practice on the part of both Americans and Ugandans. The intense focus on the individual self-management of disease is obviously limited in scope by certain structural factors—for instance, poverty, gender inequality, and domestic violence. Certain populations will never be "empowered" to make the healthiest decisions and avoid disease without broader social changes that permit their empowerment. But there is also a deeper tension at the heart of the message of accountability. Its success was limited to the ways it was made to fit within other experiences for understanding health and moral behavior. This synergy was unstable, and as prone to exacerbate the differences between accountability and other Ugandan models for moral behavior as it was to alleviate these tensions.

The antihomosexuality controversy I discussed in chapter 6 highlights some of the limitations of accountability and in so doing emphasizes how indigenous categories for personhood, justice, and equality need to be made more central to projects of democratization, rights-based activism, and—most notably—global health. The rejection of the concept of gay rights by some Ugandans points to a deep dissatisfaction with certain aspects of the discourse of accountability (the intense focus on individual self-management and self-actualization), especially when such a discourse seeks to directly challenge alternative modes of moral authority. Whereas abstinence was a message that in practice allowed youth to reflect on and meet the competing moral values of interdependence and autonomy that coexited in contemporary Uganda, the idea of sexual rights, for many, seemed incompatible with Ugandan experiences of morality and self-actualization. The controversy over homosexuality, with its intense rejection of a particular rubric for sexual personhood animated by the values of personal autonomy and independence, underscores

Beyond the Accountable Subject

the fragility of accountability as a universal model for behavior and social change.

Perhaps one of the more disconcerting effects of the adoption of PEPFAR in Uganda was how the emphasis on abstinence and faithfulness worked to overlook and in many ways counteract previously successful community-based prevention strategies such as the expansion of grassroots activism and the political mobilization of women. As I noted in chapter 1, Uganda's success with AIDS prevention in the 1980s and 1990s was due not only to the popularity of the phrase "abstain and be faithful"; it also had much to do with striking changes in the political and social environment in southern Uganda, and especially the expansion of the political rights of women and the support of community-based political and social organizations. The intense focus on individual empowerment and personal accountability largely overlooks these sorts of social and structural components to social change. It also overlooks the specific ways a society considered the threat of AIDS and the ways Ugandans evaluated their own sexual behaviors and risks early on.

During the final years of my research at UHC, in 2010 and 2011, the congregation seemed deeply disillusioned by the changing cycles of international donor interest. There was resentment in the way Pastor Thomas Walusimbi spoke about the American backlash against the Anti-Homosexuality Bill and the withdrawal of financial donations the church experienced in the wake of its public support of it. For youth who had been so energized by the fight to promote abstinence there was confusion over the disconnect they saw between the earlier support by Americans for abstinence and a current era when "human rights" seemed to be the new buzzword and "sexual morality" no longer a phrase on the U.S. president's lips. My visits to UHC in recent years have provided a window onto the vagaries of international funding and the boom-and-bust cycles that define the small grants upon which many African nongovernmental organizations depend. For all of the money that was behind PEPFAR ($1 billion earmarked for "abstinence and faithfulness" prevention programs alone), from the point of view of one small-scale grantee there seemed no lasting evidence of that particular stream of money. One discouraging effect of the emphasis on accountability as an approach to prevention may be the way it did little to transform the underlying problems that contribute to HIV risk in Uganda—issues of gender inequality, access to education, and poverty. What was left in its wake was only a sense of confusion on the part of youth who had once considered themselves partners in an American project to prevent HIV/AIDS.

The story I began this book with was the story of the Ugandan "miracle"—the dramatic reversal of the epidemic that Uganda experienced in the late 1980s and early 1990s; the marked drop in HIV prevalence placed Uganda at the forefront of AIDS research and made President Yoweri Museveni a hero in the world of global health. Ugandans had succeeded in the fight against HIV/AIDS during a period when the international community was doing little to respond to the epidemic in Africa. PEPFAR's prevention policies were in part couched in terms of this earlier success, but despite the privileged place of Ugandans in the story of the policy's beginnings, PEPFAR did little to overturn the entrenched inequalities between Africans and Westerners that underlie many global health projects today. I have focused in my analysis on the effects of accountability as a particular discourse about health. But accountability also exposes some of the problems with how projects of global health are structured and implemented. In the years following PEPFAR's introduction, Uganda's AIDS prevention success was framed in terms of the personal behavior of Ugandans; they were singled out as good subjects for American compassion, good examples of accountability's reach. In this narrative, the story of the agency of Ugandan politicians and scientists was replaced by one about the behaviors and attitudes of individual Ugandans. This is another shortcoming of the emphasis on accountability in global health projects: in its emphasis on personal conduct, accountability de-emphasizes practices of knowledge production and political organizing in places like Uganda. The story of Uganda's dramatic success becomes less about a country's ability to create a scientific, political, and bureaucratic infrastructure to address disease and more about the "will" of individual Ugandans who made themselves into good subjects of global care. This is an approach that has done little to address the "paradox of inequality" at the center of global health: the ways in which dominant approaches to humanitarianism frame Africans as passive recipients of aid even as these same models attempt to "empower" needy subjects.[2]

Accountability as a mode of thinking about the self and imagining social change seemed to have established roots in Uganda. The young people I have described throughout this book clearly understood this message and many of its implications; they embraced the language of "intentionality" and "self-control." What I have tried to highlight in these pages are the ways its adoption is colored by a complex matrix of histories and cultural attitudes. Without recognition of the deeper meanings attributed to these practices in Uganda, advocates for "accountable" projects are likely to miss the diverse

Beyond the Accountable Subject

orientations toward sexuality and health that influence young people's engagement with these messages. The apparent "universality" of the "accountable subject"—the ways accountability seemed on the surface to be so easily embraced and so familiar in the eyes of American observers—is misleading. The pursuit of health in Uganda is shaped by multiple cultural orientations to the self, and restricted by clear structural inequalities. The dominance of the accountable subject in global health projects only works to obscure, rather than reveal and build upon, the diversity of these human experiences.

NOTES

Introduction

1. John Iliffe, *The African AIDS Epidemic: A History* (Oxford: James Currey, 2006), 24.

2. Justin O. Parkhurst, "Evidence, Politics and Uganda's HIV Success: Moving Forward with ABC and HIV Prevention," *Journal of International Development* 23, no. 2 (2011): 242. Parkhurst discusses some of the debates regarding data collection and early estimates of much higher national prevalence rates in the country. In the capital of Kampala, rates reported were much higher than in rural areas, which comprise the majority of Uganda's population. Urban bias in data collection may have skewed early national peak prevalence estimates to 18 percent or higher. For instance, among women attending urban antenatal clinics, rates peaked above 25 percent in 1991. For another discussion of historic prevalence rates see: Rand L. Stoneburner and Daniel Low-Beer, "Population-Level HIV Declines and Behavioral Avoidance in Uganda," *Science* 304, no. 5671 (2004): 714–15.

3. Anna Tsing, *In the Realm of the Diamond Queen: Marginality in an Out-of-the-Way Place* (Princeton, NJ: Princeton University Press, 1993). Tsing uses this phrase to highlight the assumptions Westerners hold about those who live in supposedly isolated corners of the globe, and to emphasize how such locales, far from being removed from cosmospolitan politics, are places deeply shaped by their engagement with regional and global realms.

4. President Bush used these phrases during a graduation speech at the Coast Guard Academy in 2003. See "Commencement Address at the United States Coast Guard Academy in New London, Connecticut, May 21, 2003," http://www.gpo.gov/fdsys/pkg/PPP-2003-book1/html/PPP-2003-book1-doc-pg518-3.htm.

5. Pam Das, "Is Abstinence-Only Threatening Uganda's HIV Success Story?," *Lancet Infectious Diseases* 5, no. 5 (2005): 263–64; Brooke Schoepf, "Museveni's Other War: Condoms in Uganda," *Review of African Political Economy* 31, no. 100 (2004): 372–76.

6. Human Rights Watch, "The Less They Know, the Better: Abstinence-Only HIV/AIDS Programs in Uganda," http://hrw.org/reports/2005/uganda0305/; "Is It Churlish to Criticise Bush over His Spending on AIDS?" *Lancet* 364, no. 9431 (2004): 303–4.

7. Barbara Cruikshank, *The Will to Empower: Democratic Citizens and Other Subjects* (Ithaca, NY: Cornell University Press, 1999).

8. As I note in the following chapter, images and anecdotes of African suffering figured prominently in Bush's speeches introducing the PEPFAR program.

9. Here I am referencing the title of James Ferguson's now classic study of the development apparatus in Lesotho, as well as later work by anthropologists Miriam Ticktin and China Scherz. They point to the ways the fields of humanitarianism and development claim politically neutral, "antipolitical" stances and in so doing obscure how such work as often reinforces and reproduces forms of gendered, racial, and economic inequality. James Ferguson, *The Anti-Politics Machine: Development, Depoliticization, and Bureaucratic Power in Lesotho* (Minneapolis: University of Minnesota Press, 1994); Miriam Ticktin, *Casualties of Care: Immigration and the Politics of Humanitarianism in France* (Berkeley: University of California Press, 2011), 19; China Scherz, *Having People, Having Heart: Charity, Sustainable Development, and the Problems of Dependence in Central Uganda* (Chicago: University of Chicago Press, 2014).

10. Tania Li, *The Will to Improve: Governmentality, Development, and the Practice of Politics* (Durham, NC: Duke University Press, 2007).

11. Neil Kodesh, *Beyond the Royal Gaze: Clanship and Public Healing in Uganda* (Charlottesville: University of Virginia Press, 2010), 181.

12. Li, *The Will to Improve*. "The will to improve" is a phrase coined by Tania Li to highlight some of the same shifts in international governance and development that I also emphasize.

13. This "faith" in an individual's capacity for change was seen most obviously in the stipulation that abstinence and faithfulness be assured of one-third of prevention-related funding. But it was also evident in more insidious regulations, such as the requirement that recipients of all PEPFAR grants sign a pledge that they will not promote or advocate sex trafficking or prostitution. Such a requirement was meant to limit prostitution (and the exploitation of women many American legislators associate with sex work), but it did so by expressly restricting grant recipients' abilities to serve this population of women. Women were encouraged to change their behaviors, but were expressly given no other forms of structural support to enable them to do so. The onus on change was purposefully located and limited to women's internalized choices and removed from the broader economic and social contexts in which those choices were made and constrained.

14. James Ferguson, "The Uses of Neoliberalism," *Antipode* 41, no. s1 (2010): 166–84; Daniel Mains, "Blackouts and Progress: Privatization, Infrastructure, and the Developmentalist State in Jimma, Ethiopia." *Cultural Anthropology* 27, no. 1 (2012): 3–27.

15. Nikolas Rose, *Powers of Freedom: Reframing Political Thought* (Cambridge: Cambridge University Press, 1999); Aihwa Ong, *Neoliberalism as Exception: Mutations in Citizenship and Sovereignty* (Durham, NC: Duke University Press, 2006); Daromir Rudnyckyj, *Spiritual Economies: Islam, Globalization, and the Afterlife of Development* (Ithaca, NY: Cornell University Press, 2010).

16. Michel Foucault, *The Birth of Biopolitics: Lectures at the College de France, 1978–1979*, trans. Graham Burchell (New York: Palgrave Macmillan, 2008).

17. David Harvey, *A Brief History of Neoliberalism* (Oxford: Oxford University Press, 2005), 7.

18. Rose, *Powers of Freedom*, 141.

19. See Li, *The Will to Improve*; Harri Englund, *Prisoners of Freedom: Human Rights and the African Poor* (Berkeley: University of California Press, 2006); and Julia Paley, *Marketing Democracy: Power and Social Movements in Post-Dictatorship Peru* (Berkeley: University of California Press, 2001).

20. Rudnyckyj, *Spiritual Economies*, 4.

21. Foucault, *The Birth of Biopolitics*.

22. Adriana Petryna, *Life Exposed: Biological Citizens after Chernobyl* (Princeton, NJ: Princeton University Press, 2003); Vinh-Kim Nguyen, *The Republic of Therapy: Triage and Sovereignty in West Africa's Time of AIDS* (Durham, NC: Duke University Press, 2010).

23. Nikolas Rose, *The Politics of Life Itself* (Princeton, NJ: Princeton University Press, 2007).

24. Ben Jones, *Beyond the State in Rural Uganda* (Edinburgh: Edinburgh University Press, 2009), 2; Joseph Tumushabe, *The Politics of HIV/AIDS in Uganda*, Social Policy and Development Paper no. 28 (Geneva: United Nations Research Institute for Social Development, 2006), 5.

25. Katharina Hofer, "The Role of Evangelical NGOs in International Development: A Comparative Case Study of Kenya and Uganda," *Africa Spectrum* 38, no. 3 (2003): 385.

26. Ibid.

27. Petryna, *Life Exposed*; Erica Caple James, *Democratic Insecurities: Violence, Trauma, and Intervention in Haiti* (Berkeley: University of California Press, 2010); Nguyen, *The Republic of Therapy*; Ticktin, *Casualties of Care*; Andrea Muehlebach, *The Moral Neoliberal: Welfare and Citizenship in Italy* (Chicago: University of Chicago Press, 2012).

28. Nguyen, *The Republic of Therapy*, 6.

29. Adriana Petryna, "Experimentality: On the Global Mobility and Regulation of Human Subjects Research," *PoLAR* 30, no. 2 (2007).

30. Karen Booth, *Local Women, Global Science: Fighting AIDS in Kenya* (Bloomington: Indiana University Press, 2004); Adriana Petryna, *When Experiments Travel: Clinical Trials and the Global Search for Human Subjects* (Princeton, NJ: Princeton University Press, 2009); Nguyen, *The Republic of Therapy*.

31. Stephen Feierman, "Struggles for Control: The Social Basis of Health and Healing in Africa," *African Studies Review* 28, nos. 2–3 (1985): 73–147; Kodesh, *Beyond the Royal Gaze*.

32. Kodesh, *Beyond the Royal Gaze*, 16.

33. E. E. Evans-Pritchard, *Witchcraft, Oracles and Magic among the Azande* (Oxford: Oxford University Press, 1976); Feierman, "Struggles for Control"; Susan Whyte, *Questioning Misfortune: The Pragmatics of Uncertainty in Eastern Uganda* (Cambridge: Cambridge University Press, 1998); Julie Livingston, *Debility and the Moral Imagination in Botswana* (Bloomington: Indiana University Press, 2005).

34. One major distinction is the types of evidence and systems of knowledge Western "public health" programs and older systems of public healing draw upon. Julie Livingston elaborates on such distinctions in *Debility and the Moral Imagination*, 16–18.

35. Livingston, *Debility and the Moral Imagination*, 21.

36. T. O. Beidelman, *Moral Imagination in Kaguru Modes of Thought* (Washington, DC: Smithsonian Institution Press, 1986).

37. Beidelman, *Moral Imagination*, 2; see also Arthur Kleinman, *Living a Moral Life amidst Uncertainty and Danger* (Oxford: Oxford University Press, 2007).

38. Livingston, *Debility and the Moral Imagination*, 20.

39. For examples of studies that consider moral conflict at the center of broader experiences of social change, see Livingston, *Debility and the Moral Imagination*; Sherine Hamdy, *Our Bodies Belong to God: Organ Transplants, Islam, and the Struggle for Human Dignity in Egypt* (Berkeley: University of California Press, 2012); Joel Robbins, *Becoming Sinners: Christianity and Moral Torment in a Papua New Guinea Society* (Berkeley: University of California Press, 2004); Jennifer Cole, *Sex and Salvation: Imagining the Future in Madagascar* (Chicago: University of Chicago Press, 2010); and John Barker, "Introduction," in *The Anthropology of Morality in Melanesia and Beyond*, ed. John Barker (New York: Ashgate, 2007), 1–21.

40. Laura Deeb, *An Enchanted Modern: Gender and Public Piety in Lebanon* (Princeton, NJ: Princeton University Press, 2006); Saba Mahmood, *Politics of Piety: The Islamic Revival and the Feminist Subject* (Princeton, NJ: Princeton University Press, 2005); Charles Hirschkind, *The Ethical Soundscape: Cassette Sermons and Islamic Counterpublics* (New York: Columbia University Press, 2006); Robbins, *Becoming Sinners*; Webb Keane, *Christian Moderns: Freedom and Fetish in the Mission Encounter* (Berkeley: University of California Press, 2007); Birgit Meyer, *Translating the Devil: Religion and Modernity among the Ewe of Ghana* (Trenton, NJ: Africa World Press, 1999).

41. Meyer, *Translating the Devil*.

42. There are clearly exceptions in the ethnographic record concerning the discontinuity associated with religious conversion and other forms of radical social change. Joel Robbins's study of a Papua New Guinean society's engagement with Christianity provides one of the most cogent and insightful examples of what he calls the "moral torment" that conflicts between competing social value systems may provoke; see Robbins, *Becoming Sinners*.

43. See Cole, *Sex and Salvation*, 5.

44. Michel Foucault, "Technologies of the Self," in *Technologies of the Self: A Seminar with Michel Foucault*, ed. Luther H. Martin, Huck Gutman, and Patrick H. Hutton (Amherst: University of Massachusetts Press, 1988), 16–49; see also James Laidlaw, "For an Anthropology of Ethics and Freedom," *Journal of the Royal Anthropological Institute* 8, no. 2 (2002): 311–32; Mahmood, *Politics of Piety*.

45. Several recent ethnographies have focused attention on the specific moral orientations attributed to projects such as human rights and "development" and the ways dominant frameworks of liberal social action—autonomy, individual agency, even "freedom" itself—often obscure alternative ethical practices, coexisting within communities, which engender different relationships between self and authority, action and embodiment. See, for instance: Mahmood, *Politics of Piety*, 38; Talal Asad, *Formations of the Secular: Christianity, Islam, Modernity* (Stanford, CA: Stanford University Press, 2003); Englund, *Prisoners of Freedom*; Laidlaw, "For an

Anthropology of Ethics and Freedom"; Li, *The Will to Improve*; and Paley, *Marketing Democracy*.

46. Hansorg Dilger, "'We Are All Going to Die': Kinship, Belonging, and the Morality of HIV/AIDS-Related Illnesses and Deaths in Rural Tanzania," *Anthropological Quarterly* 81, no. 1 (2008): 207–32.

47. Heike Behrend, "The Rise of Occult Powers: AIDS and the Roman Catholic Church in Western Uganda," *Journal of Religion in Africa* 37, no. 1 (2007): 41–58.

48. Charles Piot, *Nostalgia for the Future: West Africa after the Cold War* (Chicago: University of Chicago Press, 2010), 9; see also Achille Mbembe, *On the Postcolony* (Berkeley: University of California Press, 2001); and Ruth Marshall, *Political Spiritualities: The Pentecostal Revolution in Nigeria* (Chicago: University of Chicago Press, 2009).

49. Omri Elisha, *Moral Ambition: Mobilization and Social Outreach in Evangelical Megachurches* (Berkeley: University of California Press, 2011).

50. Ibid., 18.

51. Derek R. Peterson, *Ethnic Patriotism and the East African Revival: A History of Dissent, c. 1935–1972* (Cambridge: Cambridge University Press, 2012), 281.

52. See, for instance, Elisha, *Moral Ambition*; Jeff Sharlet, *The Family: The Secret Fundamentalism at the Heart of American Power* (New York: HarperCollins, 2009); and Faye Ginsburg, *Contested Lives: The Abortion Debate in an American Community* (Berkeley: University of California Press, 1986).

53. The Baganda are the people (Muganda, singular) who historically have lived in the region around Kampala. Buganda is their kingdom and region, Luganda their language. In the Luganda language adjectives take different prefixes depending on the nouns they modify. Because of this there is no consistent adjectival form to describe things and people from the region. I will use "Ganda," the root with no prefix, throughout the book.

54. Informant confidentiality was part of the human subjects protocol approved for this study and discussed and agreed upon with interviewees. In an effort to best ensure informant privacy, the names of churches have also been changed.

55. Geertz, Clifford. "Thick Description: Toward an Interpretive Theory of Culture," in *The Interpretation of Cultures* (New York: Basic Books, 1973): 3–32.

56. Susan Harding, *The Book of Jerry Falwell: Fundamentalist Language and Politics* (Princeton, NJ: Princeton University Press, 2001).

57. Susan Harding, "Representing Fundamentalism: The Problem of the Repugnant Cultural Other," *Social Research* 58, no. 2 (1991): 373–93.

58. Catrin Evans and Helen Lambert, "Implementing Community Interventions for HIV Prevention: Insights from Project Ethnography," *Social Science and Medicine* 66, no. 2 (2008): 469. See also Shanti Parikh, "'They Arrested Me for Loving a Schoolgirl': Ethnography, HIV, and a Feminist Assessment of the Age of Consent Law as a Gender-Based Structural Intervention in Uganda," *Social Science and Medicine* 74, no. 11 (2012): 1774–82.

59. The Anti-Homosexuality Bill briefly became law in 2014 before being annulled by the high court of Uganda. The annulment did not address the content of

the bill, but ruled that the bill had not been properly voted on by the parliament and was therefore not legal.

Chapter 1: American Compassion and the Politics of AIDS Prevention in Uganda

1. Jennifer Brier, *Infectious Ideas: U.S. Political Responses to the AIDS Crisis* (Chapel Hill: University of North Carolina Press, 2011), 80.

2. For a nuanced history of the Reagan administration's approach to the AIDS epidemic see Brier, *Infectious Ideas*, chapter 3.

3. Katherine Q. Seelye, "Helms Puts the Brakes to a Bill Financing AIDS Treatment," *New York Times*, July 5, 1995.

4. Ibid. It is worth noting that the Ryan White Act was passed after its namesake had become widely known by Americans. White was a hemophiliac who was infected via a blood transfusion in the years before blood banks screened for HIV; his image as an "innocent" victim is widely acknowledged to have elicited a sea change in public perceptions of the AIDS epidemic. As is evident in the act's name, his case was instrumental in garnering public support for the financing of AIDS programs.

5. George W. Bush, "President Delivers 'State of the Union,'" http://george wbush-whitehouse.archives.gov/news/releases/2003/01/20030128-19.html.

6. Several Christian missionary groups were involved in AIDS orphan work and orphan sponsorship programs, but their advocacy for people living with AIDS, and their work in the AIDS education sector, was far more limited prior to the advent of PEPFAR.

7. Christine J. Gardner, *Making Chastity Sexy: The Rhetoric of Evangelical Abstinence Campaigns* (Chicago: University of Chicago Press, 2011), 145.

8. The faith-based initiative program, a focus of the early Bush administration, was intended to facilitate the distribution of federal funding to religious and community organizations and to foster greater involvement of religious organizations in policy making.

9. These policy changes were deeply controversial not only for the general American public but also for evangelical and conservative Christian communities. The faith-based initiative program existed alongside Charitable Choice, a Bush era welfare program that was intended to expand the number of religious organizations competing for federal grants; both were criticized for creating a vague relationship of oversight between the government and religious entities. Secular critics complained that such policies allowed for proselytizing, though work explicitly devoted to promoting particular religious beliefs was still considered unconstitutional. In the religious sector such policies stoked fears that federal funding would result in new forms of governmental regulation that many Christian organizations found objectionable. See Omri Elisha, *Moral Ambition: Mobilization and Social Outreach in Evangelical Megachurches* (Berkeley: University of California Press, 2011).

10. Bush, "President Delivers 'State of the Union.'"

11. See Jim A. Kuypers et al., "Compassionate Conservatism: The Rhetorical Reconstruction of Conservative Rhetoric," *American Communication Journal* 6, no. 4 (2003): 1–27.

12. In one of his first acts as president, Bush outlined his faith-based initiative in a policy document circulated to Congress and titled *Rallying the Armies of Compassion* (House Document 107–36).

13. Barbara Cruikshank, *The Will to Empower: Democratic Citizens and Other Subjects* (Ithaca, NY: Cornell University Press, 1999); Donna Goldstein, "Microenterprise Training Programs, Neoliberal Common Sense, and the Discourses of Self-Esteem," in *The New Poverty Studies: The Ethnography of Power, Politics, and Impoverished People in the United States*, ed. Judith Goode and Jeff Maskovsky (New York: New York University Press, 2001), 236–72; Sandra Morgan and Jeff Maskovsky, "The Anthropology of Welfare 'Reform': New Perspectives on U.S. Urban Poverty in the Post-Welfare Era," *Annual Review of Anthropology* 32 (2003): 315–38.

14. David Harvey, *The Condition of Postmodernity* (New York: Blackwell, 1989); Cruikshank, *The Will to Empower*.

15. Cruikshank, *The Will to Empower*; Edith Archambault and Judith Boumendil, "Dilemmas of Public/Private Partnership in France," in *Dilemmas of the Welfare Mix: The New Structure of Welfare in an Age of Privitization*, ed. Ugo Ascoli and Costanzo Ranci (New York: Springer, 2002), 109–34; Morgan and Maskovsky, "The Anthropology of Welfare 'Reform'"; Julia Paley, *Marketing Democracy: Power and Social Movements in Post-Dictatorship Peru* (Berkeley: University of California Press, 2001); Erica Bornstein, *Disquieting Gifts: Humanitarianism in New Delhi* (Stanford, CA: Stanford University Press, 2012); Andrea Muehlebach, *The Moral Neoliberal: Welfare and Citizenship in Italy* (Chicago: University of Chicago Press, 2012).

16. Muehleback, *The Moral Neoliberal*.

17. Ibid., 11.

18. Ibid.

19. Marcel Mauss, *The Gift: The Form and Reason for Exchange in Archaic Societies* (New York: Norton, 2000).

20. Miriam Ticktin, *Casualties of Care: Immigration and the Politics of Humanitarianism in France*, (Berkeley: University of California Press, 2011).

21. Erica James, *Democratic Insecurities: Violence, Trauma, and Intervention in Haiti* (Berkeley: University of California Press, 2010), 85.

22. Ticktin, *Casualties of Care*.

23. Ibid., 3; Adriana Petryna, *Life Exposed: Biological Citizens after Chernobyl* (Princeton, NJ: Princeton University Press, 2003); Vinh-Kim Nguyen, *The Republic of Therapy: Triage and Sovereignty in West Africa's Time of AIDS* (Durham, NC: Duke University Press, 2010); James, *Democratic Insecurities*.

24. See Nguyen, *The Republic of Therapy*.

25. 107th Congress, 1st Session, House Document 107–36, "Rallying the Armies of Compassion," 4.

26. Ibid., 6–7.

27. Elisha, *Moral Ambition*, 155.

28. Elisha, *Moral Ambition*.

29. Ibid.

30. United Nations General Assembly Special Session on HIV/AIDS, "Statement Delivered by Peter Piot, Executive Director, UNAIDS," June 25, 2001, http://www .un.org/ga/aids/statements/docs/Piot25JuneFINAL.htm.

31. John W. Dietrich, "The Politics of PEPFAR: The President's Emergency Plan for AIDS Relief," *Ethics and International Affairs* 21, no. 3 (2007): 277–92.

32. The Brazilian program has been widely celebrated for providing ARV treatment to all citizens regardless of their ability to pay.

33. Ticktin, *Casualties of Care*; Nguyen, *The Republic of Therapy*.

34. Targeted nations for PEPFAR I (2003–8) were Botswana, Côte d'Ivoire, Ethiopia, Guyana, Haiti, Kenya, Mozambique, Namibia, Nigeria, Rwanda, South Africa, Tanzania, Uganda, Vietnam, and Zambia.

35. Raymond W. Copson, "AIDS in Africa," in *AIDS in Africa: A Pandemic on the Move*, ed. Garson Claton (Hauppauge, NY: Nova Science, 2006), 21. These numbers include smaller U.S. programs run separately from PEPFAR; PEPFAR funds alone accounted for just over $1.2 billion. Before the creation of PEPFAR, USAID directly administered most funds for AIDS programs. The government now has a dedicated office at the Department of State to administer PEPFAR funds, the Global HIV/ AIDS Initiative. USAID continues to have a smaller budget for its own dedicated AIDS initiatives.

36. Government of Uganda, *UNGASS Country Progress Report Uganda, January 2006 to December 2007* (Geneva, Switzerland: WHO, 2008), 31.

37. Besides the restrictions on prevention programs discussed here, other controversial aspects of the first iteration of PEPFAR (2003–8) included restrictions on treating women in the sex industry and the denial of access to generic ARV drugs. Active sex workers were prohibited from being the focus of funded programs, and had to sign a pledge promising not to participate in the sex industry if they were to receive treatment or care. PEPFAR has also been accused of limiting access to (easier, cheaper) generic ARV therapies in favor of brand-name ARVs; see Copson, "AIDS in Africa," 20. But PEPFAR's prevention constraints have drawn the most vociferous complaints.

38. "Is It Churlish to Criticise Bush over His Spending on AIDS?" *Lancet* 364, no. 9431 (2004): 303.

39. As with domestic welfare reform, the Bush administration had altered federal policy so as to permit and encourage religious organizations to receive funding for administering federal programs, including PEPFAR.

40. "Is It Churlish to Criticise Bush over His Spending on AIDS?"

41. Teresa Swezey and Michele Teitelbaum, "HIV/AIDS and the Context of Polygyny and Other Marital and Sexual Unions in Africa: Implications for Risk Assessment and Interventions," in *AIDS, Culture, and Africa*, ed. Douglas Feldman (Gainesville: University of Florida Press, 2008), 231; Human Rights Watch, "The Less They Know, the Better: Abstinence-Only HIV/AIDS Programs in Uganda," http:// hrw.org/reports/2005/uganda0305/; Steven Sinding, "Does 'CNN' (Condoms,

Needles and Negotiation) Work Better than 'ABC' (Abstinence, Faithfulness and Condom Use) in Attacking the AIDS Epidemic?" *International Family Planning Perspectives* 31, no. 1 (2005): 38–40; James Putzel, "The Politics of Action on AIDS: A Case Study of Uganda," *Public Administration and Development* 24, no. 1 (2004): 19–30.

42. Dr. Sinding served as director-general of the International Planned Parenthood Federation from 2002 to 2006. He published his evaluation of the abstinence and faithfulness strategy in 2005; see Sinding, "Does 'CNN' Work Better than 'ABC'?"

43. Yoweri Museveni, "Behavioral Change Is the Only Way to Fight AIDS," *Wall Street Journal*, July 14, 2004; http://www.ph.ucla.edu/epi/seaids/behavioralchange.html.

44. Andrew Mwenda, "Uganda's Politics of Foreign Aid and Violent Conflict: The Political Uses of the LRA Rebellion," in *The Lord's Resistance Army: Myth and Reality*, ed. Tim Allen and Koen Vlassenroot, (London: Zed, 2010), 45–54.

45. Joseph Tumushabe, *The Politics of HIV/AIDS in Uganda* (Geneva: United Nations Research Institute for Social Development, 2006), 5.

46. Katharina Hofer, "The Role of Evangelical NGOs in International Development: A Comparative Case Study of Kenya and Uganda," *Africa Spectrum* 38, no. 3 (2003): 375–98.

47. For an account of these shifts in international aid, see Daniel Jordan Smith, *A Culture of Corruption: Everyday Deception and Popular Discontent in Nigeria* (Princeton, NJ: Princeton University Press, 2008), 97.

48. Cruikshank, *The Will to Empower*, 4.

49. See Yoweri Museveni, *Sowing the Mustard Seed: The Struggle for Freedom and Democracy in Uganda* (New York: Macmillan Educational, 1997); and Yoweri Museveni, *What Is Africa's Problem?* (Minneapolis: University of Minnesota Press, 1992). See also Nelson Kasfir, "Guerrillas and Civilian Participation: The National Resistance Army in Uganda, 1981–86," *Journal of Modern African Studies* 43, no. 2 (2005): 276.

50. Museveni was critical of multiparty politics because he argued that it intensified ethnic and religious divisions in the country. Criticisms of Museveni grew before the 2006 elections, when he pressured the courts to overturn constitutional term limits so that he could seek a third term after twenty years in power. He also jailed his main opponent under suspicion of treason, thereby limiting his opponent's ability to campaign. Museveni easily won reelection, though there were sporadic riots in Kampala and in the east and north, areas where support for Museveni was weakest. Political opposition to his rule has grown in recent years and the protection of civil liberties—particularly freedom of the press—has been repeatedly curtailed by the Museveni government.

51. Wendy Stokes, *Women in Contemporary Politics* (Cambridge: Polity, 2005), 170.

52. In 1981 there was only one woman representative in Uganda's parliament; by 2001 the parliament comprised nearly 25 percent women.

53. In recent years criticism has escalated of the NRM leadership and Museveni regarding women's rights. Toward the late 1990s, momentum in the women's movement seemed to have slowed, with more resistance from higher levels of

government; see Anne Marie Goetz, "No Shortcuts to Power: Constraints on Women's Political Effectiveness in Uganda," *Journal of Modern African Studies* 40, no. 4 (2002): 549–75. For a fuller analysis of gender and politics in Uganda, including criticisms of Museveni's policies toward women, see Sylvia Tamale, *When Hens Begin to Crow: Gender and Parliamentary Politics in Uganda* (Boulder, CO: Westview, 1999).

54. Robert Thornton, *Unimagined Community: Sex, Networks, and AIDS in Uganda and South Africa* (Berkeley: University of California Press, 2008), 19.

55. Douglas Kirby and David Halperin, "Success in Uganda: An Analysis of Behavior Changes that Led to Declines in HIV Prevalence in the Early 1990s," cited in Justin O. Parkhurst, "Evidence, Politics and Uganda's HIV Success: Moving Forward with ABC and HIV Prevention," *Journal of International Development* 23, no. 2 (2011), 243.

56. Thornton, *Unimagined Community*, 19.

57. Edward C. Green et al., "Uganda's HIV Prevention Success: The Role of Sexual Behavior Change and the National Response," *AIDS and Behavior* 10, no. 4 (2006): 342.

58. Daniel Low-Beer and Rand Stoneburner, "Behaviour and Communication Change in Reducing HIV: Is Uganda Unique?," *African Journal of AIDS Research* 2, no. 1 (2003): 9–10.

59. James Putzel, "The Politics of Action on AIDS: A Case Study of Uganda," *Public Administration and Development* 24, no. 1 (2004): 19–30.

60. John Kinsman, *AIDS Policy in Uganda: Evidence, Ideology, and the Making of an African Success Story* (New York: Palgrave Macmillan, 2010), 71.

61. Susan Cohen, "Beyond Slogans: Lessons from Uganda's Experience with ABC and HIV/AIDS," *Reproductive Health Matters* 12, no. 23 (2004): 132–35; Robinah Mirembe, "AIDS and Democratic Education in Uganda," *Comparative Education* 38, no. 3 (2002): 291–302; Green et al., "Uganda's HIV Prevention Success."

62. Thornton, *Unimagined Community*, 19.

63. Hearing before the House Subcommittee on Health, "HIV/AIDS, TB, and Malaria: Combating a Global Pandemic" 108th Congress, 1st Session. U.S. Government Printing Office Serial no. 108-10, March 20, 2003. The bill being discussed is H.R. 1298, "The United States Leadership against HIV/AIDS, Tuberculosis and Malaria Act of 2003." This bill authorized $15 billion for unilateral and bilateral spending on AIDS, an authorization that made the PEPFAR program possible.

64. Ibid., 5.

65. Ibid., 32.

66. Brooke Schoepf, "Museveni's Other War: Condoms in Uganda," *Review of African Political Economy* 31, no. 100 (2004): 372–76.

67. These were two of the terms PEPFAR administrators used to classify programs, determine the allocation of aid (especially given that a percentage of program funds were reserved for "abstain and be faithful"), and measure program efficacy and reach. I take up the effects of this kind of program disaggregation in more detail in the next section of this chapter.

68. Hearing before the Senate Subcommittee on African Affairs, "Fighting AIDS in Uganda: What Went Right?" 108th Congress, 1st Session. U.S. Government

Printing Office, S. Hrg. 108-106, May 19, 2003, 12. Claude Allen, deputy director of Health and Human Services under Bush, made similar references to the Ugandan culture of abstinence and faithfulness in his statements before the House subcommittee on health, a hearing referenced above, in March 2003; see House Hearing "HIV/AIDS, TB, and Malaria," 18.

69. Helen Epstein, *The Invisible Cure: Africa, the West, and the Fight against AIDS* (New York: Farrar, Straus and Giroux, 2007); Thornton, *Unimagined Community*; Timothy L. Mah and Daniel Halperin, "Concurrent Sexual Partnerships and the HIV Epidemic in Africa: Evidence to Move Forward," *AIDS and Behavior* 14, no. 1 (2010): 11–16.

70. For a discussion of the structural and political changes that contributed to Uganda's prevention success, see Elaine Murphy et al., "Was the ABC Approach (Abstinence, Being Faithful, Using Condoms) Responsible for Uganda's Decline in HIV?" *PLoS Medicine* 3, no. 9 (2006): e379.

71. Epstein, *The Invisible Cure*, 194.

72. An example is the quote from Janet Museveni cited by Anne Peterson in a Senate hearing: "How are we going to teach children to be law-abiding citizens if we do not train them to exercise self-control and to learn to police themselves while they are still young and teachable? Not to guide our young in this way implies that we as adults and leaders have no faith in human nature and in our ability as beings to exercise self-control. If this is the case, then we are surely a doomed species"; see "Fighting AIDS in Uganda," S. Hrg. 108–106, 14.

73. Oliver Duff, "Public Health and Religion: AIDS, America, Abstinence," *Independent* (United Kingdom), June 1, 2006. Straight Talk Uganda has since reincorporated information about condom use into some of its programs. Given the Ugandan government's strong support of PEPFAR's guidelines, the pressure that some long-term programs felt to convert to an abstinence-only message was likely considerable.

74. Human Rights Watch, *The Less They Know the Better*, 1.

75. U.S. President's Emergency Plan for AIDS Relief, *Fiscal Year 2005 Operational Plan, June 2005 Update* (Washington, DC: Office of the United States Global AIDS Coordinator, 2005), 109.

76. PEPFAR has been criticized for a lack of transparency in partner selection. However, the PEPFAR website provides lists of primary and secondary program partners for the years 2004–7; see United States President's Emergency Plan for AIDS Relief, "Uganda—Partners," http://www.pepfar.gov/countries/c19720.htm.

77. Helen Epstein reported that the Children's AIDS Fund received an "unfit" rating on its first proposal for PEPFAR funds in 2004, but the project was funded despite this, most likely under pressure from the Bush administration, which had personal ties to the Smiths; see Epstein, *The Invisible Cure*, 302.

78. Two of the churches where I spent time, University Hill Church (UHC) and another that I refer to as Central Kampala Church, received funds indirectly from PEPFAR. In both cases an intermediary NGO (and not the church directly) received program funds, and the church managed and hosted the AIDS prevention project that was being funded. In the case of UHC, the NGO was a subsidiary of

the church itself, and the management of the NGO and the church were deeply intertwined. PEPFAR grants were usually administrated via a multitiered system, with "prime" partners directly receiving funds from the U.S. government and contracting out work to subpartners. Grants at the subpartner level could be quite modest. For instance, in 2005, UHC's NGO received a grant of less than ten thousand dollars to manage a youth abstinence education program.

79. This percentage is for all programs, including the 80 percent of programming primarily focused on treatment. If more than one program area is listed, it is not clear from the information available what percentage a particular grant recipient devotes to each program area it lists.

80. United States President's Emergency Plan for AIDS Relief, *Uganda Fiscal Year 2008 PEPFAR Country Operational Plan (COP)*, http://www.pepfar.gov/about /opplan08/102010.htm.

Chapter 2: AIDS at Home

1. The legacy of a devastating twenty-year civil war in northern Uganda continues to destabilize that region. See Sverker Finnström, *Living with Bad Surroundings: War, History, and Everyday Moments in Northern Uganda* (Durham, NC: Duke University Press, 2008); and Heike Behrend, *Alice Lakwena and Holy Spirits: War in Northern Uganda, 1986–97* (Athens: Ohio University Press, 2000) for ethnographic accounts.

2. Edward C. Green and Allison Herling Ruark, *AIDS Behavior and Culture: Understanding Evidence-Based Prevention* (Walnut Creek, CA: Left Coast, 2011), 12; Helen Epstein, *The Invisible Cure: Africa, the West, and the Fight against AIDS* (New York: Farrar, Straus and Giroux, 2007), 169.

3. Derek Peterson, *Ethnic Patriotism and the East African Revival: A History of Dissent, c. 1935–1972* (Cambridge: Cambridge University Press, 2012), 17.

4. The term *ekitiibwa* is usually translated as either "respect" or "honor." Historian John Iliffe's essay on honor in Buganda provides an overview of the meaning of this term in the kingdom prior to and during the early colonial period; see John Iliffe, "Ekitiibwaa and Martyrdom," in *Honour in African History* (Cambridge: Cambridge University Press, 2004), 161–80. In chapter 3, I discuss how ekitiibwa shaped sexual attitudes and behaviors.

5. Shane Doyle, "Premarital Sexuality in Great Lakes Africa, 1900–1980," in *Generations Past: Youth in East African History*, ed. Andrew Burton and Helene Charton-Bigot (Athens: Ohio University Press, 2010), 241.

6. Nakanyike Musisi, "Women, 'Elite Polygyny,' and Buganda State Formation," *Signs* 16, no. 4 (1991): 757–86. Grace Bantebya Kyomuhendo and Marjorie Keniston McIntosh, *Women, Work and Domestic Virtue in Uganda (1900–2003)* (Oxford: Currey, 2006).

7. Miriam Goheen, *Men Own the Fields, Women Own the Crops: Gender and Power in the Cameroon Grasslands* (Madison: University of Wisconsin Press, 1996); Judith van Allen, "Sitting on a Man: Colonialism and the Lost Political Institutions of Igbo Women," *Canadian Journal of African Studies* 6, no. 2 (1972): 165–81.

8. Lucy Mair, *An African People in the Twentieth Century* (New York: Russell and Russell, 1934), 59.

9. Ibid., 50.

10. Holger Bernt Hansen, *Mission, Church, and State in a Colonial Setting: Uganda, 1890–1925* (New York: St. Martin's, 1984), 280; Mikael Karlström, "Modernity and Its Aspirants: Moral Community and Development Eutopianism in Buganda," *Current Anthropology* 45, no. 4 (2004): 601.

11. Under the terms of British indirect rule, both customary law and British common law was upheld. Africans were typically subject to customary law, but in the instance of marriage, monogamous marriages were validated by the church and held to the terms of British marriage statutes. Anglican missionaries had won this concession from the state early on; see Hansen, *Mission, Church, and State*, 67. Today Ugandan marriages may be legally recognized through multiple channels: in a customary manner, which usually demands participation in a cultural ceremony (most often, a bridewealth exchange); through a Christian or Muslim wedding; or, least commonly, by registering the marriage in a state court.

12. "Marriage of Natives in Uganda 1938," digest of replies to questionnaire accompanying chief secretary's circular No. D. 177/1/61 of April 19, 1938, on native marriage, Church of Uganda Provincial Archives, Bp 178.1005, 10.

13. "Marriage of Natives in Uganda 1931," reply to questionnaire on native marriage in Uganda, Church of Uganda Provincial Archives, Bp 178.1006, 3.

14. See Nakanyike Musisi, "Morality as Identity: the Missionary Moral Agenda in Buganda, 1877–1945," *Journal of Religious History* 23, no. 1 (1999): 51–74. Unlike other historical narratives of early missionary efforts (in Africa and elsewhere), the existence of a court society that engaged religion as a new form of power and influence also meant that early converts in Buganda were often drawn from the elite rather than from socially vulnerable populations (e.g., widows and orphans). Elsewhere such populations pursued religious conversion as a desirable alternative to a social system that marginalized them; see Doyle, "Premarital Sexuality in Great Lakes Africa," 243. Religion was recognized early on as form of power and status, though not necessarily a stable, uncontested one. For accounts of religious change in late-nineteenth-century Buganda, see D. A. Low, *Buganda in Modern History* (Berkeley: University of California Press, 1971); and C. C. Wrigley, "The Christian Revolution in Buganda," *Comparative Studies in Society and History* 2, no. 1 (1959): 33–58.

15. Nakanyike Musisi, "Gender and the Cultural Construction of 'Bad Women' in the Development of Kampala-Kibuga, 1900–1962," in *"Wicked" Women and the Reconfiguration of Gender in Africa*, ed. Dorothy L. Hodgson and Sheryl A. McCurdy (Portsmouth, NH: Heinemann, 2001), 171–87.

16. Ganda petitioner, quoted in Peterson, *Ethnic Patriotism*, 96.

17. "Marriage of Natives in Uganda 1931," letter from the bishops house convening a conference on marriage and issues relating to the new marriage ordinance, Church of Uganda Provincial Archives, Bp 178.1006, 15–16.

18. Holly Hanson, *Landed Obligation: The Practice of Power in Buganda* (Portsmouth, NH: Heinemann, 2003). Private landownership—a right selectively bestowed

on loyal Christian chiefs under the 1900 Uganda Agreement—proved especially controversial and, as Hanson argues, its introduction likely played a major part in stoking the pervading sense of moral crisis that defined this period. Land had long been central to virtually all social and political relationships in Buganda, and its sudden transformation into a commodity was blamed for the emergence of numerous new social problems: the "disobedience" of a new class of renters, the "abusive" tendencies of new landlords, and the monetization of bridewealth and the ensuing independence of youth from the control of their elders that this enabled. See Hanson, *Landed Obligation*, 216–26; see also Karlström, "Modernity and Its Aspirants," 601.

19. Peterson, *Ethnic Patriotism*, 96.

20. Ibid., 97. Peterson notes that the focus on fidelity and virginity was a "convenient fiction" that had little basis in actual patterns of Ganda intimate relationships, "traditional" or otherwise.

21. Hanson, *Landed Obligation*, 1.

22. Most famously, Kabaka Mwanga had sex with young male pages, causing much consternation among missionaries, an issue I return to in chapter 6. Men with great power were permitted sexual relationships that exceeded the terms of what were considered normative sexual relationships. The power to break these rules of behavior reflected, and reinforced, their own status and distinction.

23. Musisi, "Women, 'Elite Polygyny,' and State Formation."

24. Karlström, "Modernity and Its Aspirants," 600.

25. Jesumi Miti, quoted in Peterson, *Ethnic Patriotism*, 96.

26. Peterson, *Ethnic Patriotism*, 97.

27. A. W. Southall and P. C. W. Gutkind, *Townsmen in the Making: Kampala and Its Suburbs* (Kampala, Uganda: East African Institute for Social Research, 1957).

28. Such partnerships continue to be very common in Kampala. See Paula Jean Davis, "On the Sexuality of 'Town Women' in Kampala," *Africa Today* 47, no. 3 (2000): 28–61; and Jessica A. Ogden, "'Producing' Respect: The 'Proper Woman' in Postcolonial Kampala," in *Postcolonial Identities in Africa*, ed. R. P. Werbner and T. O. Ranger (New York: Zed, 1996), 165–92.

29. This category of partnership, while drawing on the descriptive terms of European romantic love and friendship, closely resembles the precolonial category of *bakirerese* (restless) women who traveled to find short-term domestic partners but who were considered morally suspect for doing so. See Davis, "On the Sexuality of 'Town Women'"; and Christine Obbo, "Dominant Male Ideology and Female Options: Three African Case Studies," *Africa* 46, no. 4 (1976): 371–89.

30. Lucy Mair, *African Marriage and Social Change* (London: Cass, 1969), 71.

31. Peterson, *Ethnic Patriotism*, 49.

32. While unsolicited public accounting of personal misconduct would have been highly unusual, accusations of sexual misconduct were used as a political strategy in precolonial Buganda. See Apolo Kagwa, *The Kings of Buganda*, trans. M. S. M. Kiwanuka (Nairobi, Kenya: East African Publishing House, 1971), 10.

33. Derek Peterson, "Wordy Women: Gender Trouble and the Oral Politics of the East African Revival in Gikuyuland," *Journal of African History* 42, no. 3 (2001): 469–89.

34. Carol Summers, "Grandfathers, Grandsons, Morality, and Radical Politics in Late Colonial Buganda," *International Journal of African Historical Studies* 38, no. 3 (2005): 430.

35. See, for example, Adam Ashforth, *Witchcraft, Violence, and Democracy in South Africa* (Chicago: University of Chicago Press, 2005); Deborah Posel, "The Scandal of Manhood: 'Baby Rape' and the Politicization of Sexual Violence in Post-Apartheid South Africa," *Culture, Health and Sexuality* 7, no. 3 (2005): 239–52; Louise Vincent, "Virginity Testing in South Africa: Re-traditioning the Postcolony," *Culture, Health and Sexuality* 8, no. 1 (2006): 17–30.

36. Betty Iyamuremye, "Marriage and Divorce Bill to Protect Marriages," *New Vision* (Uganda), March 19, 2013, http://www.newvision.co.ug/news/640829 -marriage-and-divorce-bill-to-protect-marriages.html. Muslims were exempt from the new bill because of a 2008 law that relegated all Muslim marital, inheritance, and family disputes to a special Quadi Muslim court.

37. Haji Nsereko Mutumba, "Loopholes in the Marriage and Divorce Bill," *New Vision* (Uganda), April 2, 2013, http://www.newvision.co.ug/news/641265-loopholes -in-the-marriage-and-divorce-bill.html.

38. "Born-again" is the term most commonly used by Ugandans to describe nonmainline charismatic churches; it includes but is not limited to those that identify as Pentecostal. Such charismatic churches are distinguished by their emphasis on experiential salvation, being "born again" in Christ, and their belief in a literal reading of the Bible. In Uganda and much of sub-Saharan Africa they are also associated with a cosmopolitan worldview, one that is expressed through both personal relationships with Christians abroad and through a symbolic emphasis on internationalism. Use of media, music, and technology also differentiates these churches, especially from mainline churches that often follow a common liturgy and, in the Anglican Church, still sing from hymnals published in the late nineteenth century.

39. In addition to the Marriage and Divorce Bill there has been the Anti-Homosexuality Bill, which I discuss in chapter 6, as well as a new public decency law, commonly refered to as the "miniskirt ban," that has sought to curb both pornography and women's "indecent" clothing.

40. Ruth Marshall, *Political Spiritualities: The Pentecostal Revolution in Nigeria* (Chicago: University of Chicago Press, 2009), 46.

41. Omri Elisha, *Moral Ambition: Mobilization and Social Outreach in Evangelical Megachurches* (Berkeley: University of California Press, 2011).

42. Work on charismatic and Pentecostal Christianity in recent years has focused on its global connections, and the similarities of styles of worship among diverse local communities; see David Lehmann, *Struggle for the Spirit: Religious Transformation and Popular Culture in Brazil and Latin America* (Cambridge: Blackwell, 1996); David Lyon, *Jesus in Disneyland: Religion in Postmodern Times* (Cambridge: Polity, 2000); and

Simon Coleman, *The Globalisation of Charismatic Christianity: Spreading the Gospel of Prosperity* (Cambridge: Cambridge University Press, 2000). Other work on non-mainline Christianity theorized its popularity in part because it provided an alternative network of relationships that competed with the dominance of traditional kin groups; see Elizabeth Brusco, *The Reformation of Machismo: Evangelical Conversion and Gender in Colombia* (Austin: University of Texas Press, 1995); Lesley Gill, "'Like a Veil to Cover Them': Women and the Pentecostal Movement in La Paz," *American Ethnologist* 17, no. 4 (1990): 709–21; and Stephen Hunt, "'Neither Here nor There': The Construction of Identities and Boundary Maintenance of West African Pentecostals," *Sociology* 36, no. 1 (2002): 146–69. It was thus set against "traditional" modes of authority and dominance, proving particularly attractive for women and young men.

43. Jane Guyer and Samuel Belinga, "Wealth in People as Wealth in Knowledge: Accumulation and Composition in Equatorial Africa," *Journal of African History* 36, no. 1 (1995): 93–94.

44. See Neil Kodesh, *Beyond the Royal Gaze: Clanship and Public Healing in Uganda* (Charlottesville: University of Virginia Press, 2011); and Summers, "Grandfathers, Grandsons."

Chapter 3: "Abstinence Is for Me, How about You?"

1. See Helen Epstein, *The Invisible Cure: Africa, the West, and the Fight against AIDS* (New York: Farrar, Straus and Giroux, 2007), 190, for one account of this pledge. Muwenda Mutebi II is the current king, or *kabaka*, of Buganda, a constitutional kingdom within the nation of Uganda. In the early 1990s President Yoweri Museveni sought to restore the Ugandan traditional kingdoms of the African Great Lakes region as important cultural institutions. These kingdoms had earlier been dissolved under President Milton Obote because they were viewed as political threats to national leaders in the period following independence.

2. These studies argue that prevention programs that only emphasize individual decision making (i.e., "Just say no!") obscure the social and economic contexts that shape sexual relationships. When a girl must decide whether to drop out of school or exchange sex for the school fees that keep her enrolled, the choice to abstain becomes more complicated than a simple evaluation of self-control. This dilemma becomes starker in the face of data that show that girls who drop out of school are at higher risk of marrying young and at greater risk of HIV infection. On structural risk see, for instance, Catherine Campbell, *Letting Them Die: Why HIV Prevention Programs Fail* (Oxford: Currey, 2003); Maryinez Lyons, "Mobile Populations and HIV/AIDS in East Africa," in *HIV and AIDS in Africa: Beyond Epidemiology*, ed. Ezekiel Kalipeni, Susan Craddock, Joseph R. Oppong, and Jayati Gosh (Malden, MA: Blackwell, 2004), 175–90; Geeta Rao Gupta et al., "Structural Approaches to HIV Prevention," *Lancet* 372, no. 9640 (2008): 764–75; Shanti Parikh, "The Political Economy of Marriage and HIV: The ABC Approach, 'Safe' Infidelity, and Managing Moral Risk in Uganda," *Framing Health Matters* 97, no. 7 (2007), 1198–99; and Esther Sumartojo, "Structural Factors in HIV Prevention: Concepts, Examples, and Implications for Research," *AIDS* 14, suppl. 1 (2000): S3–10.

3. This dedication to promoting abstinence was by no means unique. Churches similar to UHC—located in Kampala's city center and catering to urban youth—were broadly invested in promoting abstinence and marital faithfulness during the years of my fieldwork. The radio station run by another church—one of the larger Christian radio stations in Kampala—regularly held high school and university outreach events, hosted by their DJs, that took up the topic of youth sexuality. Missionary groups visiting Kampala, and hosted by local churches, periodically ran abstinence education workshops (one of which I discuss later in this chapter), and gave visiting lectures to congregations on the topic of AIDS prevention. This is to say that UHC was but one of several churches that had embraced this issue and that promoted it with vigor to Kampala's youth population.

4. For accounts of this shift: David Martin, *Pentecostalism: The World Their Parish* (Oxford: Blackwell, 2002); Philip Jenkins, *The Next Christendom: The Coming of Global Christianity* (Oxford: Oxford University Press, 2002); Joel Robbins, "The Globalization of Charismatic and Pentecostal Christianity," *Annual Review of Anthropology* 33 (2004), 117–43.

5. Simon Coleman, *The Globalisation of Charismatic Christianity: Spreading the Gospel of Prosperity* (Cambridge: Cambridge University Press, 2000), 34.

6. Jeff Sharlet, *The Family: Power, Politics and Fundamentalism's Shadow Elite* (New York: HarperCollins, 2009), provides more information about the organization that runs the National Prayer Breakfast and the international political reach of that organization's American evangelical founders.

7. The PEPFAR grants Walusimbi received through his church's NGO were not large enough to sustain the church (nor were they intended to) and were earmarked for particular education projects that were discontinued when funding ran out.

8. For instance, one individual American had pledged two thousand dollars per month to the church for a set period to support student programs and internships. Another church in the United States had a long-term relationship with UHC, helping with both direct financial pledges and with the funding of larger independent projects such as conferences and AIDS education events that UHC helped to host and run. Many of these financial relationships were cultivated when foreign Christians came and visited Uganda, seeking out Ugandan congregations and Christian programs to support. This was a fairly common way that Ugandan churches, especially urban, English speaking congregations accessible to American visitors, might garner foreign support and connections. (Short-term mission trips abroad, often lasting the length of an American vacation, have become commonplace in many American evangelical congregations.) While such relationships were not institutionalized in any way at UHC, they were a frequent, though sometimes intermittent and unpredictable, source of support for the congregation. The importance of these relationships was emphasized to me when I returned in 2010 and the church was suffering from the withdrawal of many of these small sponsorship arrangements in the wake of the fallout from Uganda's 2009 Anti-Homosexuality Bill (a controversy I discuss in chapter 6). That year Robert, the church manager, worried aloud to me about the future of the church, complaining that it was not able to survive on the weekly tithes and pledges of church members. He told me that the church's

"building fund" collection plate, meant to support rent and related expenses, often received no more than forty thousand Ugandan shillings (about US$20) each week, a sum that was far too small to cover church expenses.

9. I should emphasize that while Pastor Walusimbi was clearly adept at drawing in foreign financial backing for his church he also cultivated his independence from American donors. This was at no time more apparent than in the wake of the controversy stemming from the Anti-Homosexuality Bill, a period during which he was resolute in his support of the controversial bill even as American donors withdrew their financial support (see note 8, above).

10. Mahmood Mamdani, *Scholars in the Marketplace: The Dilemmas of Neo-liberal Reform at Makerere University, 1989–2005* (Dakar, Senegal: CODESRIA, 2007). Mamdani's incisive account of these transformations notes that humanities departments were encouraged during these years to "take any Arts subject, [and] join it with a skill in demand" so that "Religious Studies" became "Religious Studies and Conflict Resolution" and "Geography" became "Geography and Tourism" (53).

11. Jean Comaroff and John Comaroff, "Millennial Capitalism and the Culture of Neoliberalism," *Public Culture* 12, no. 2 (2000): 291–343.

12. Daromir Rudnyckyj, *Spiritual Economies: Islam, Globalization, and the Afterlife of Development* (Ithaca, NY: Cornell University Press, 2010).

13. Faramerz Dabhoiwala, *The Origins of Sex: A History of the First Sexual Revolution* (Oxford: Oxford University Press, 2012).

14. Ibid., 87.

15. For further discussion of the concept of Christian personhood, see Louis Dumont, "A Modified View of Our Origins: The Christian Beginnings of Modern Individualism," *Religion* 12, no.1 (1982): 1–27. For a broader review of Western constructions of the "individual" in European and American philosophy and political thought, see Rosalind Shaw, "'Tok Af, Lef Af': A Political Economy of Temne Techniques of Secrecy and Self," in *African Philosophy as Cultural Inquiry*, ed. Ivan Karp and D. A. Masolo (Bloomington: Indiana University Press, 2000), 26–29; and, for a more thorough discussion of the topic, Charles Taylor, *The Sources of the Self: The Making of the Modern Identity* (Cambridge, MA: Harvard University Press, 1989). For a discussion of the limitations of the association of individualism with modern Protestant Christianity, see Omri Elisha, *Moral Ambition: Mobilization and Social Outreach in Evangelical Megachurches* (Berkeley: University of California Press, 2011), 21.

16. Webb Keane, *Christian Moderns: Freedom and Fetish in the Mission Encounter* (Berkeley: University of California Press, 2007), 51.

17. Talal Asad, *Formations of the Secular: Christianity, Islam, Modernity* (Stanford, CA: Stanford University Press, 2003); Harri Englund, *Prisoners of Freedom: Human Rights and the African Poor* (Berkeley: University of California Press, 2006); Saba Mahmood, *Politics of Piety: The Islamic Revival and the Feminist Subject* (Princeton, NJ: Princeton University Press, 2005); Nikolas Rose, *The Politics of Life Itself* (Princeton, NJ: Princeton University Press, 2007).

18. Placide Tempels, *Bantu Philosophy* (Paris: Presence Africaine, 1959); John Mbiti, *African Religions and Philosophy* (London: Heinemann, 1992); Godfrey Lienhardt, "Self: Public and Private—Some African Representations," in *The Category*

of the Person: Anthropology, Philosophy, History, ed. Michael Carrithers, Steven Collins, and Steven Lukes (Cambridge: Cambridge University Press, 1985); Edward LiPuma, "Modernity and Forms of Personhood in Melanesia," in *Bodies and Persons: Comparative Perspectives from Africa and Melanesia*, ed. Michael Lambek and Andrew Strathern (Cambridge: Cambridge University Press, 1998); Elisha, *Moral Ambition*, 20.

19. Charles Piot, *Remotely Global: Village Modernity in West Africa* (Chicago: University of Chicago Press, 1999), 18.

20. The study of "occult economies" in Africa and scholarship that has sought to theorize and understand the "modernity of witchcraft" provide rich analyses of the moral struggles stoked by economic changes that have challenged these models of personhood and put them in direct conflict with a Western emphasis on the individual subject. Capital accumulation has especially driven such rebukes, where individual wealth accumulation that is not reinvested in socially productive relationships is viewed as spiritually dangerous and morally threatening. See, for instance, Peter Geschiere, *The Modernity of Witchcraft: Politics and the Occult in Postcolonial Africa* (Charlottesville: University of Virginia Press, 1997); and Henrietta Moore and Todd Sanders, eds., *Magical Interpretations, Material Realities: Modernity, Witchcraft and the Occult in Postcolonial Africa* (London: Routledge, 2001).

21. James Laidlaw, "For an Anthropology of Ethics and Freedom," *Journal of the Royal Anthropological Institute* 8, no. 2 (2002), 311–32; see also Keane, *Christian Moderns*, 52.

22. See Mahmood, *Politics of Piety*, 38.

23. Suzette Heald, "The Power of Sex: Some Reflections of the Caldwells' 'African Sexuality' Thesis," *Africa* 65, no. 4 (1995): 496; see also T. O. Beidelman, *The Cool Knife: Imagery of Gender, Sexuality and Moral Education in Kaguru Initiation* (Washington, DC: Smithsonian Institution Press, 1997).

24. John Iliffe, "Ekitiibwaa and Martyrdom," in *Honour in African History* (Cambridge: Cambridge University Press, 2004), 161–80.

25. Samuel Kasule, "Popular Performance and the Construction of Social Reality in Post-Amin Uganda," *Journal of Popular Culture* 32, no. 2 (1998): 49.

26. See Ruth Mukama, "Women's Discourses as the Conservators of Cultural Values in Language," *International Journal of the Sociology of Language* 129, no. 1 (1998), 157–66.

27. See Shanti Parikh, "From Auntie to Disco: The Bifurcation of Risk and Pleasure in Sex Education in Uganda," in *Sex in Development: Science, Sexuality and Morality in Global Perspective*, ed. Vincanne Adams and Stacy Leigh Pigg (Durham, NC: Duke University Press, 2005), 131.

28. Suzette Heald, *Manhood and Morality: Sex, Violence and Ritual in Gisu Society* (New York: Routledge, 1999), 141.

29. Pastor Walusimbi is referring to the fact that during Ganda traditional marriage ceremonies, *kwanjula*, a female goat, is usually given by the groom's family to the bride's. It is meant, in some interpretations, to represent the bride's virginity and to thus honor her parents for "raising her well."

30. Museveni trained and was educated in Dar es Salaam during the *Ujamma* reforms, and his early approach to governance is generally interpreted as being shaped

by socialist principles. Walusimbi is referring to this popular reading of Museveni's early political views.

31. Lessons followed Growing Kids God's Way, an American Christian curriculum series. The pastors who led the session used textbooks and videos distributed by the U.S. Christian publisher Biblical Ethics for Parenting; they had acquired these materials when they spent a year living in the United States.

32. Emily Martin, *Flexible Bodies: The Role of Immunity in American Culture from the Days of Polio to the Age of AIDS* (Boston: Beacon, 1994). Martin's study of American metaphors for disease focuses on the emergence of a discourse about "flexible bodies" in the United States during the 1990s; it may also resonate with the contemporary discussions of disease and self-sufficiency during the neoliberal era in Uganda that I have outlined here.

33. Jo Sadgrove, "'Keeping Up Appearances': Sex and Religion amongst University Students in Uganda," *Journal of Religion in Africa* 37, no. 1 (2007): 116–44; Alessandro Gussman, "HIV/AIDS, Pentecostal Churches, and the Joseph Generation in Uganda," *Africa Today* 56, no. 1 (2009): 67–86.

Chapter 4: Abstinence and the Healthy Body

1. Emily Martin, *Flexible Bodies: The Role of Immunity in American Culture from the Days of Polio to the Age of AIDS* (Boston: Beacon, 1994), 243.

2. Claire L. Wendland, *A Heart for the Work: Journeys through an African Medical School* (Chicago: University of Chicago Press, 2010), 17.

3. Martin's focus in *Flexible Bodies* on narrative and symbolic representations of illness reflects the influence of an early strand of medical anthropology often associated with the work of Arthur Kleinman and the broader field of phenomenology, which focused on the ways people make sense of illness and how such "interpretive practices" and shared symbolic meanings helped shape intersubjective states and experiences of the body that in turn demand certain responses or forms of therapeutic attention. See Byron Good, *Medicine, Rationality and Experience: An Anthropological Perspective* (Cambridge: Cambridge University Press, 1994).

4. Jean Comaroff, "Healing and the Cultural Order: The Case of the Barolong boo Ratshidi," *American Ethnologist* 7, no. 4 (1980): 639, quoted in Matthew Engelke, *The Problem of Presence: Beyond Scripture in an African Church* (Berkeley: University of California Press, 2007), 230.

5. Neil Kodesh, *Beyond the Royal Gaze: Clanship and Public Healing in Uganda* (Charlottesville: University of Virginia Press, 2010), 181.

6. Susan Reynolds Whyte, *Questioning Misfortune: The Pragmatics of Uncertainty in Eastern Uganda* (Cambridge: Cambridge University Press, 1998), 30.

7. This is an idea traced in other studies of health and illness on the African continent—especially those that focus on the ways witchcraft becomes a framework through which to understand and address physical illness. See, for instance, Adam Ashforth, *Witchcraft, Violence, and Democracy in South Africa* (Chicago: University of Chicago Press, 2005); Alexander Rödlach, *Witches, Westerners, and HIV: AIDS and Cultures of Blame in Africa* (Walnut Creek, CA: Left Coast, 2006).

8. See Stephen Feierman, *Health and Society in Africa: A Working Bibliography* (Honolulu, HI: Crossroads Press, 1979); and Stephen Feierman, "Struggles for Control: The Social Basis of Health and Healing in Africa," *African Studies Review* 28, nos. 2–3 (1985): 73–147. For discussions of the role of health as an aspect of the colonial endeavor, and its effects on African subjectivity see: Jean Comaroff, *Body of Power, Spirit of Resistance: The Culture and History of a South African People* (Chicago: University of Chicago Press, 1985); Jean Comaroff and John Comaroff, *Of Revelation and Revolution*, vol. 1, *Christianity, Colonialism, and Consciousness in South Africa* (Chicago: University of Chicago Press, 1997); Nancy Rose Hunt, *A Colonial Lexicon: Of Birth Ritual, Medicalization, and Mobility in the Congo* (Durham, NC: Duke University Press, 1999); and Jonathan Sadowsky, *Imperial Bedlam: Institutions of Madness in Colonial Southwest Nigeria* (Berkeley: University of California Press, 1999).

9. Whyte, *Questioning Misfortune*, 3.

10. Julie Livingston, *Debility and the Moral Imagination in Botswana* (Bloomington: Indiana University Press, 2005), 3.

11. Susan Whyte's book is an excellent study of the ways Ugandans view biomedicine as one form of healing that is complimentary to, rather than in opposition with, traditional medicine (Whyte, *Questioning Misfortune*). Her work demonstrates the ways that moral and physical insecurity drives the pursuit of multiple forms of therapy in communities with limited access to biomedical care. Stacey Langwick's study of traditional healing in Tanzania similarly explores the coexistence of biomedical and other forms of health care in an African community. Stacey Langwick, *Bodies, Politics and African Healing: The Matter of Maladies in Tanzania* (Bloomington: Indiana University Press, 2011).

12. There is a wide range of Christian articulations of the spirit-versus-body dichotomy. See Fenella Cannell, "The Christianity of Anthropology," in *The Anthropology of Christianity*, ed. Fenella Cannell (Durham, NC: Duke University Press, 2005), 1–50; and Frederick Klaits, *Death in a Church of Life: Moral Passion during Botswana's Time of AIDS* (Berkeley: University of California Press, 2010).

13. Thomas Csordas, *The Sacred Self: A Cultural Phenomenology of Charismatic Healing* (Berkeley: University of California Press, 1997), 3.

14. Kodesh, *Beyond the Royal Gaze*, 15.

15. See Klaits, *Death in a Church of Life*, 161; and Cannell, "The Christianity of Anthropology."

16. Livingston, *Debility and the Moral Imagination*, 4.

17. See, for instance, Peter Geschiere, *The Modernity of Witchcraft: Politics and the Occult in Postcolonial Africa* (Charlottesville: University of Virginia Press, 1997); and Henrietta Moore and Todd Sanders, eds., *Magical Interpretations, Material Realities: Modernity, Witchcraft and the Occult in Postcolonial Africa* (London: Routledge, 2001).

18. Birgit Meyer, *Translating the Devil: Religion and Modernity among the Ewe of Ghana* (Trenton, NJ: Africa World Press, 1999); Matthew Engelke, *The Problem of Presence: Beyond Scripture in an African Church* (Berkeley: University of California Press, 2007).

19. Allan Anderson, "Exorcism and Conversion to African Pentecostalism," *Exchange* 35, no. 1 (2006): 116–33; Caroline Jeannerat, "Of Lizards, Misfortune and

Deliverance: Pentecostal Soteriology in the Life of a Migrant," *African Studies* 68, no. 2 (2009): 251–71; Martin Lindhardt, "The Ambivalence of Power: Charismatic Christianity and Occult Forces in Urban Tanzania," *Nordic Journal of Religion and Society* 22, no. 1 (2009): 37–54.

20. See Whyte, *Questioning Misfortune.*

21. Feierman, "Struggles for Control," and Kodesh, *Beyond the Royal Gaze,* both reflect on the fact that fertility was a natural concern to associate with the realm of ancestral spirits because the ability to reproduce and raise socially recognized, healthy children is an issue central to the broader concerns of the family and clan. Additionally, and especially for women, reproduction was an essential part of the life cycle, necessary to become a fully adult member of society. Failure to reproduce could bring about intense scrutiny and anxiety for which spiritual mediation was usually sought. (It was a problem for men as well, but in that infertility was not understood as an embodied experience for men their unsuccessful reproduction was not as often problematized.)

22. The connection of Pastor Herman's grandmother to spirit mediumship was never made explicitly, but it is known that Ganda women who suffered from problems with fertility were frequently made candidates for mediumship. Women who did not or could not reproduce were often viewed as embodying a liminal social status that made them well suited to such work.

23. There are several precolonial kingdoms in southern Uganda, one of which was Buganda, which had royal classes of people considered to be distinct from commoners.

24. Jezebel is mentioned twice in the Bible: first in the Old Testament, in the first and second books of Kings, where she is a Phoenician princess who marries King Ahab, turning him from God and converting him to the worship of the pagan god Baal, subjecting the Hebrews to decades of sin and tyranny. In the New Testament she appears in the book of Revelation as a prophet who incites members of the church to commit acts of sexual immorality.

Chapter 5: Faithfulness

1. In particular, research has focused on the prevalence of concurrent, long-term multiple partnerships in sub-Saharan Africa and the risk they pose for HIV/AIDS transmission. John Caldwell, Pat Caldwell, and Pat Quiggin, "The Social Context of AIDS in Sub-Saharan Africa," *Population and Development Review* 15, no. 2 (1989): 185–234, highlights multiple-partner relations as one element of what the authors theorize to be a distinct African system of sexuality (in contrast to European models) that has made Africans more vulnerable to HIV/AIDS. More recent work has presented concurrent multiple partnerships not as a static model of African sexuality but as emergent from historically and culturally specific experiences that present particular challenges for HIV prevention. See Robert J. Thornton, *Unimagined Community: Sex, Networks, and AIDS in Uganda and South Africa* (Berkeley: University of California Press, 2008); Mark Hunter, "Cultural Politics and Masculinities: Multiple-Partners in Historical Perspective in KwaZulu-Natal," *Culture, Health*

and Sexuality 7, no. 4 (2005): 389–403; and Helen Epstein, *The Invisible Cure: Africa, the West, and the Fight against AIDS* (New York: Farrar, Straus and Giroux, 2007).

2. For corresponding studies on masculinity and multiple partners, see Shanti Parikh, "The Political Economy of Marriage and HIV: The ABC Approach, 'Safe' Infidelity, and Managing Moral Risk in Uganda," *Framing Health Matters* 97, no. 7 (2007): 1198–1208; and Hunter, "Cultural Politics." On HIV/AIDS risk in relation to gender, see Karen Booth, *Local Women, Global Science: Fighting AIDS in Kenya* (Bloomington: Indiana University Press, 2004).

3. A 2004 report by the Joint United Nations Programme on HIV/AIDS (UNAIDS) highlighted the fact that a growing proportion of new infections worldwide were in women, and that as high as 50 percent of recent infections in some regions were happening within marriages, between spouses; UNAIDS, *2004 Report on the Global AIDS Epidemic* (Geneva: UNAIDS, 2004), 29.

4. The idea that love is transformative of the object of affection is not limited to Christian ideologies of emotion. Frederick Klaits, in his rich study of the emotion within a Tswana community affected by HIV/AIDS, also describes the ways that the emotions of love and jealousy may affect the well-being of others. Tswana affective registers are performative and distinctly social; they are believed to shape the experience of health and the practice of care. See Frederick Klaits, *Death in a Church of Life: Moral Passion during Botswana's Time of AIDS* (Berkeley: University of California Press, 2010).

5. One need look no further than American and European public service announcements for smoking cessation; see Kim Witte and Mike Allen, "A Meta-Analysis of Fear Appeals: Implications for Effective Public Health Campaigns," *Health, Education and Behavior* 27, no. 5 (2000): 591–615.

6. George F. Lowenstein et al., "Risk as Feelings," *Psychological Bulletin* 127, no. 2 (2000): 267–86; Paul Rozin and April E. Fallon, "A Perspective on Disgust," *Psychological Review* 94, no. 1 (1987): 23–41.

7. Lori L. Heise and Christopher Elias, "Transforming AIDS Prevention to Meet Women's Needs: A Focus on Developing Countries," *Social Science and Medicine* 40, no. 7 (1995): 931–43; Parikh, "The Political Economy of Marriage."

8. Teresa Swezey and Michele Teitelbaum, "HIV/AIDS and the Context of Polygyny and Other Marital and Sexual Unions in Africa: Implications for Risk Assessment and Interventions," in *AIDS, Culture, and Africa*, ed. Douglas Feldman (Gainesville: University of Florida Press, 2008), 220–38.

9. Lynn M. Thomas and Jennifer Cole, "Thinking through Love in Africa," in *Love in Africa*, ed. Jennifer Cole and Lynn M. Thomas (Chicago: University of Chicago Press, 2009), 6.

10. Catherine Lutz, *Unnatural Emotions: Everyday Sentiments on a Micronesian Atoll and Their Challenge to Western Theory* (Chicago: University of Chicago Press, 1988), 4.

11. Lila Abu-Lughod, *Veiled Sentiments: Honor and Poetry in a Bedouin Society* (Berkeley: University of California Press, 1986); Laura M. Ahearn, *Invitations to Love: Literacy, Love Letters, and Social Change in Nepal* (Ann Arbor: University of Michigan Press, 2001); Holly Wardlow and Jennifer Hirsch, "Introduction," in *Modern Loves:*

The *Anthropology of Romantic Courtship and Companionate Marriage*, ed. Holly Wardlow and Jennifer Hirsch (Ann Arbor: University of Michigan Press, 2006): 1–34.

12. Ahearn, *Invitations to Love*, 48.

13. Thomas and Cole, "Thinking through Love in Africa," 7.

14. Ibid., 8; Megan Vaughan, *Curing Their Ills: Colonial Power and African Illness* (London: Polity, 1991).

15. Caldwell et al., "The Social Context of AIDS."

16. Suzette Heald, "The Power of Sex: Some Reflections of the Caldwells' 'African Sexuality' Thesis," *Africa* 65, no. 4 (1995): 489–505.

17. Thomas and Cole, "Thinking through Love in Africa," 15.

18. Wardlow and Hirsch, *Modern Loves*.

19. Friedrich Engels, *Origin of the Family, Private Property, and the State* (Harmondsworth, England: Penguin, 1985).

20. Lawrence Stone, *The Family, Sex, and Marriage in England, 1500–1800* (New York: Harper and Row, 1977).

21. Ahearn, *Invitations to Love*, 8.

22. A. W. Southall and P. C. W. Gutkind, *Townsmen in the Making: Kampala and Its Suburbs* (Kampala, Uganda: East African Institute for Social Research, 1957); Lucy Mair, *African Marriage and Social Change* (London: Cass, 1969).

23. For further discussion relating to South Africa, see Mark Hunter, *Love in the Time of AIDS* (Bloomington: Indiana University Press, 2010), 5.

24. For another example of such gendered modes of complaint, see Anthony Simpson, *Boys to Men in the Shadow of AIDS: Masculinities and HIV Risk in Zambia* (New York: Palgrave Macmillan, 2009).

25. Young people's portrayals of their parent's sexual relationships and attitudes are notoriously unreliable. See Kearsley Stewart, "Toward a Historical Perspective on Sexuality in Uganda: The Reproductive Lifeline Technique for Grandmothers and Their Daughters," *Africa Today* 47, nos. 3–4 (2001): 122–48. In Kampala it is likely that the conflicted attitudes about dating and romance shared by young people today were also shared by their parents twenty and thirty years ago. By the mid-twentieth century in Uganda and throughout much of the rest of urbanized Africa, companionate marriage and romantic love were common topics in music and popular culture even as marriage itself was becoming less common and informal domestic partnerships increasingly the norm. Nonetheless, the idea of "traditional" relationships is still a pervasive discourse, as I discuss later in this chapter.

26. Jean Comaroff and John L. Comaroff, "Millennial Capitalism and the Culture of Neoliberalism," *Public Culture* 12, no. 2 (2000): 291–343.

27. See, for instance, Daniel Jordan Smith, *A Culture of Corruption: Everyday Deception and Popular Discontent in Nigeria* (Princeton, NJ: Princeton University Press, 2008). Another UHC student wrote a joke online for his friends that featured ATMs and highlighted the ambiguous nature of the wealth such machines represented. He wrote, "I used to think 'getting saved' was an assured means of using my ATM often." Here ATMs represent a wealth associated with the "prosperity gospel," a Christian belief popular in Uganda and throughout the world (though not at UHC) in

which investment in the church, and reliance on faith alone, promises great material returns. The writer of the joke meant to highlight how such forms of seemingly "magical" accumulation, represented here and in the skit by an ATM, are morally ambiguous and the focus of criticism.

28. This skit took place in the wake of a series of riots in response to President Yoweri Museveni's decision to sell pristine, and traditionally sacred, forest at the edge of the Buganda kingdom to an Indian sugar processing company.

29. For other studies of urban Ugandan youth's attitudes about romance and the ways that money features prominently in discussions about intimacy and love in Uganda, see David Mills and Richard Ssewakiryanga, "'No Romance without Finance': Masculinities, Commodities and HIV in Uganda," in *Readings in Gender in Africa*, ed. Andrea Cornwall (Oxford: James Currey, 2005), 90–94; Parikh, "The Political Economy of Marriage"; and Jo Sadgrove, "'Keeping Up Appearances': Sex and Religion amongst University Students in Uganda," *Journal of Religion in Africa* 37, no. 1 (2007): 116–44.

30. The moral distinction between people and things is a long-standing tension theorized by anthropologists. Marcel Mauss's work on gift giving is central to these discussions; see Mauss, *The Gift: The Form and Reason for Exchange in Archaic Societies* (New York: Norton, 1990). Mauss's study was followed by a wealth of literature concerning theories of exchange in Melanesia; see, for example, Bronislaw Malinowski, *Argonauts of the Western Pacific* (Prospect Heights, IL: Waveland, 1984); and Annette Weiner, *Inalienable Possessions* (Berkeley: University of California Press, 1992). In Africanist literature a related debate concerning wealth and exchange is made in discussions of the prominence of the "wealth in people" system of status and accumulation (and the significance of patron clientism) that complicates clear distinctions between commodity and gift exchange. See Caroline Bledsoe, *Women and Marriage in Kpelle Society* (Stanford, CA: Stanford University Press, 1980); Jane Guyer, "Wealth in People and Self-Realization in Equatorial Africa," *Man* 28, no. 2 (1993): 243–65; and Sandra Barnes, *Patrons and Power: Creating a Political Community in Contemporary Lagos* (Manchester, England: Manchester University Press, 1986). In terms of missionary resistance to bridewealth, Webb Keane has highlighted two assumptions that Protestants made about such exchanges in Sumba, Indonesia, to bolster their arguments against such ceremonies. The first was that ceremonial exchanges produce the same alienating effects as commodity exchange, and the second that human value is derived from its very distinctiveness from—and superiority to—material things, making such exchanges immoral. See Webb Keane, *Christian Moderns: Freedom and Fetish in the Mission Encounter* (Berkeley: University of California Press, 2007), 71. Christians' and Africans' divergent views of the moral purpose and effects of exchange established long-standing tensions surrounding bridewealth, some of which I discussed in chapter 2.

31. Keane, *Christian Moderns*, 71; emphasis in the original.

32. Klaits, *Death in a Church of Life*, 4.

33. Holly Hanson, *Landed Obligation: The Practice of Power in Buganda* (Portsmouth, NH: Heinemann, 2003), 1.

34. Southall and Gutkind, *Townsmen in the Making*, 156. As I discussed in chapter 2, church marriages became status symbols for elite Ugandans early in the colonial period. By the mid-1950s, as described by Southall and Gutkind in their survey of urban life, attitudes about church weddings and other forms of marriage had transformed the ways that ordinary city dwellers considered their domestic arrangements. For a description of such transformations, see Michael Twaddle, *Kakungulu and the Creation of Uganda, 1868–1928* (London: Currey, 1993).

35. As early as the 1930s, Lucy Mair documented the prevalence of what Ugandans sometimes now derisively refer to as "co-habitation" (the practice of sharing a home without being married) in Kampala; see Mair, *African Marriage and Social Change*, 71. As I noted in chapter 2, a range of more and less formal forms of domestic unions—from "free" marriage to "friend" relationships—was documented by researchers in the city by midcentury; see Southall and Gutkind, *Townsmen in the Making*, 153–72.

36. Georg Simmel, *The Philosophy of Money*, trans. Tom Bottomore and David Frisby (London: Routledge, 1978); see also Sharon Hutchinson, "The Cattle of Money and the Cattle of Girls among the Nuer, 1930–83," *American Ethnologist* 19, no. 2 (1992): 294–316.

37. Hutchinson, "The Cattle of Money," 294.

38. See Jennifer Cole, "Fresh Contact in Tamatave, Madagascar," *American Ethnologist* 31, no. 4 (2004): 580.

39. Shanti Parikh, "Sugar Daddies and Sexual Citizenship in Uganda: Rethinking Third Wave Feminism," *Black Renaissance/Renaissance Noir* 6, no. 1 (2004): 82–107; Shanti Parikh, "Sex, Lies and Love Letters: Condoms, Female Agency, and Paradoxes of Romance in Uganda," *Agenda: African Feminisms* 62, no. 1 (2004): 2–20; Shanti Parikh, " 'Don't Tell Your Sister or Anyone That You Love Me': Considering the Effects of Adult Regulation on Adolescent Sexual Subjectivities in Uganda's Time of AIDS," in *Gender, Sexuality and HIV/AIDS: Research and Intervention in Africa*, ed. Britt Pinkowsky Tersbøl (Copenhagen: Institute of Public Health, University of Copenhagen, 2003), 53–84.

40. Webb Keane, "Sincerity, 'Modernity,' and the Protestants," *Cultural Anthropology* 17, no. 1 (2002): 65–92; Keane, *Christian Moderns*.

41. Keane, "Sincerity, 'Modernity,' and the Protestants," 83.

42. Augustine's writings on sexual morality, human will, and sin are credited for articulating much of our current understanding of Christian personhood. For one helpful discussion of some of these concepts, see Guy G. Stroumsa, "Caro salutis cardo: Shaping the Person in Early Christian Thought," *History of Religions* 30, no. 1 (1990): 25–50. See also the discussion of Augustine's "In Interiore Homine" in Charles Taylor, *The Sources of the Self: The Making of the Modern Identity* (Cambridge, MA: Harvard University Press, 1989), 127–43.

43. Though not considered ideal, delays in paying bridewealth were also common outside of the Christian community and are not new developments; see, for instance, Southall and Gutkind, *Townsmen in the Making*, 154–56.

44. Thornton, *Unimagined Community*; Epstein, *The Invisible Cure*.

1. Michel Foucault, *The History of Sexuality*, vol. 1, *An Introduction*, trans. Robert Hurley (New York: Vintage, 1978), 43.

2. Faramerz Dabhoiwala, *The Origins of Sex: A History of the First Sexual Revolution* (Oxford: Oxford University Press, 2012), 139.

3. Talal Asad, *Formations of the Secular: Christianity, Islam, Modernity* (Stanford, CA: Stanford University Press, 2003), 127–58; Harri Englund, *Prisoners of Freedom: Human Rights and the African Poor* (Berkeley: University of California Press, 2006).

4. Jeff Sharlet, "Straight Man's Burden: The American Roots of Uganda's Anti-Gay Persecution." *Harper's*, September 2010, 36–48; Josh Kron, "Resentment towards West Bolsters Uganda's New Anti-Gay Bill," *New York Times*, February 28, 2012.

5. A key insight in anthropological studies of gay, lesbian, bisexual, and transgender sexualities, in Africa and elsewhere, has been to emphasize how categories of sexual subjectivity are contested, partial, and often in tension with globalizing projects of sexual identity making; see Donald Donham, "Freeing South Africa: The 'Modernization' of Male-Male Sexuality in Soweto," *Cultural Anthropology* 13, no. 1 (1998): 3–21; Tom Boellstorff, "Between Religion and Desire: Being Muslim and Gay in Indonesia," *American Anthropologist* 107, no. 4 (2005): 575–85; and Tom Boellstorff, "Queer Studies in the House of Anthropology," *Annual Review of Anthropology* 36 (2007): 17–25.

6. The Lord's Resistance Army (LRA) is a guerrilla force that has been waging a civil war in northern Uganda for more than twenty years.

7. Sally Engel Merry, "Transnational Human Rights and Local Activism," *American Anthropologist* 108, no. 1 (2006): 38–51.

8. I refer to Luganda terminology in this section, as I have done in earlier discussions of this idea, but the issue of "respectability" came up in nearly every interview about sexuality I conducted with youth regardless of ethnicity. Attitudes about the importance of kin relationships and marriage were similarly consistent regardless of ethnic background.

9. Studies of contemporary marriage and urban romantic relationships in Africa have highlighted the endurance and moral significance of these models of kinship and lineage and the ways they shape modern experiences of love and family. See Daniel Jordan Smith, "Romance, Parenthood, and Gender in a Modern African Society," *Ethnology* 40, no. 2 (2001): 129–51; Lynn M. Thomas and Jennifer Cole, "Thinking through Love in Africa," in *Love in Africa*, ed. Jennifer Cole and Lynn M. Thomas (Chicago: University of Chicago Press, 2009), 1–30.

10. Sylvia Tamale, "Eroticism, Sensuality and 'Women's Secrets' among the Baganda: A Critical Analysis," *Feminist Africa* 5 (2005): 9–36; Suzette Heald, "The Power of Sex: Some Reflections of the Caldwells' 'African Sexuality' Thesis," *Africa* 65, no. 4 (1995): 489–505.

11. Mwanga's sexual appetite is especially famous because his relationships with young men became a sticking point between him and foreign missionaries in his

court, eventually leading to his decision to hold a mass execution of the youth who refused to disavow their Christian beliefs and continue their sexual relationships with him. Their execution is marked by a public holiday in Uganda, Uganda Martyrs Day, though the connection to same-sex acts is rarely if ever mentioned. For one of several scholarly accounts, see Neville Hoad, *African Intimacies: Race, Homosexuality, and Globalization* (Minneapolis: University of Minnesota Press, 2007).

12. A 1995 online discussion among scholars about the history of homosexuality in Uganda provides one window into debates about the foreignness of homosexual practices (see http://h-net.msu.edu/cgi-bin/logbrowse.pl?trx=vx&list=H -Africa&month=9511&week=c&msg=VHkRnJ/OuPSQlnvwvuxWoA&user= &pw=); the thread discusses etymological arguments about the origins of the word for homosexuality, *ebisiyaga*, and the ways such arguments have been used to draw associations between homosexuailty and the cultural influence of Arab traders in nineteenth-century Buganda. Several contributors to the thread note that the association between homosexuality and Arab traders was made in Ganda leader Apolo Kagwa's early ethnography of the Baganda. The claim that Arab traders introduced "sodomy" is found in Kagwa's book as part of a larger discussion of the "breakdown" of custom following Arab contact with Ganda society. See Apolo Kagwa, *The Customs of the Baganda*, trans. Ernest B. Kalibala (New York: Columbia University Press, 1934), 98.

13. Royal women in precolonial Buganda were similarly freed from the restrictions on sexual behavior levied on common women. Nakanyike Musisi argues that such freedoms were permitted because they helped strengthen existing social hierarchies and hegemonic gender relations; see Musisi, "Women, 'Elite Polygyny,' and Buganda State Formation," *Signs* 16, no. 4 (1991): 774.

14. Mikael Karlström, "Imagining Democracy: Political Culture and Democratisation in Buganda," *Africa* 66, no. 4 (1996): 486; Robert Wyrod, "Between Women's Rights and Men's Authority: Masculinity and Discourses of Gender Difference in Urban Uganda," *Gender and Society* 22, no. 6 (2008): 799–823.

15. Karlström, "Imagining Democracy," 486.

16. See Paula Jean Davis, "On the Sexuality of 'Town Women' in Kampala," *Africa Today* 47, no. 3 (2000): 28–61; Nakanyike Musisi, "Gender and the Cultural Construction of 'Bad Women' in the Development of Kampala-Kibuga, 1900–1962," in *"Wicked" Women and the Reconfiguration of Gender in Africa*, ed. Dorothy L. Hodgson and Sheryl A. McCurdy (Portsmouth, NH: Heinemann, 2001), 171–87.

17. For a discussion of Uganda, see Wyrod, "Between Women's Rights and Men's Authority"; for discussions of Africa more generally, see Mark Epprecht, "The Unsaying of Indigenous Homosexualities in Zimbabwe: Mapping a Blindspot in an African Masculinity," *Journal of Southern African Studies* 24, no. 4 (1998): 631–51; and Daniel Smith, "Romance, Parenthood, and Gender in a Modern African Society."

18. Martin Ssempa, "Homosexuality Is against Our Culture," *New Vision* (Uganda), September 5, 2007, reprinted in *Homosexuality: Perspectives from Uganda*, ed. Sylvia Tamale (Kampala, Uganda: Sexual Minorities of Uganda, 2007): 41–44.

19. Youth often attend church separately from their parents, especially with the proliferation of born-again congregations that cater to a younger demographic.

20. Herbert Ssempogo, "Religious Groups Demonstrate against Homosexuals," *New Vision* (Uganda), August 21, 2007.

21. Paul Kiwuuwa, "Homosexual Admits Recruiting Students." *New Vision* (Uganda), March 23, 2009.

22. "Aggravated defilement" is another category of sexual offense, introduced in the 2009 revision to the Defilement Law, which addresses the sexual abuse of minors. It stipulates that HIV-positive persons who have sex with minors are subject to the death penalty.

23. This information was revealed in the U.S. diplomatic cables made public through WikiLeaks. This cable, and one other concerning the bill, are available through the *Guardian* at http://www.guardian.co.uk/world/us-embassy-cables -documents.

24. Sylvia Tamale also notes the use of the term *recruitment* during a backlash against homosexuality in Uganda in 2003. Sylvia Tamale, "Out of the Closet: Unveiling Sexuality Discourses in Uganda," in *Africa after Gender?*, ed. Catherine M. Cole, Takyiwaa Manuh, and Stephan F. Miescher (Bloomington: Indiana University Press, 2007), 18.

25. It is important to note that this woman, and other interviewees, may not be as concerned with same-sex acts as long as those forms of sexual activity do not challenge what they view as a fundamental linking of sex, gender, and kinship. Donald Donham notes a similar disconnect between homosexual identity as it is claimed in transnational gay rights movements and local understandings of sexuality and sexual identity in South Africa. See Donham, "Freeing South Africa."

26. Periodic media coverage of child abduction and ritual murder both reflects and stokes such concerns. See also Karlström, "Modernity and Its Aspirants: Moral Community and Development Eutopianism in Buganda," *Current Anthropology* 45, no. 4 (2004): 595–610.

27. At 2011 exchange rates, this comes to less than ten U.S. cents; the monetary amount was employed to emphasize economic desperation.

28. The large literature on the "modernity" of witchcraft analyzes similar concerns about the disavowal of relationships of obligation in the pursuit of wealth. See, for instance, Birgit Meyer and Peter Pels, eds. *Magic and Modernity: Interfaces of Revelation and Concealment* (Stanford, CA: Stanford University Press, 2003); and Harry West and Todd Sanders, *Transparency and Conspiracy: Ethnographies of Suspicion in the New World Order* (Durham, NC: Duke University Press, 2003).

29. Kiwuuwa, "Homosexual Admits Recruiting Students."

30. Daniel Jordan Smith, *A Culture of Corruption: Everyday Deception and Popular Discontent in Nigeria* (Princeton, NJ: Princeton University Press, 2008), 155; Luise White, *Speaking with Vampires: Rumor and History in Colonial Africa* (Berkeley: University of California Press, 2000).

31. Sylvia Tamale, "Out of the Closet: Unveiling Sexuality Discourses in Uganda," in *Africa after Gender?*, ed. Catherine M. Cole, Takyiwaa Manuh, and Stephan F. Miescher (Bloomington: Indiana University Press, 2007), 17–29; Isak Niehaus, "Perversion of Power: Witchcraft and the Sexuality of Evil in the South African Lowveld," *Journal of Religion in Africa* 32, no. 3 (2002): 288.

32. This goal was shared with me in an interview with a pastor who said he helped draft the bill. The bill does enumerate sexual activities in detail, providing a sort of "definition" of homosexuality.

33. Georg Simmel, "The Sociology of Secrecy and Secret Societies," trans. Albion W. Small, *American Journal of Sociology* 11, no. 4 (1906).

34. Achille Mbembe, *On the Postcolony* (Berkeley: University of California Press, 2001), 144.

35. T. O. Beidelman, "The Filth of Incest: A Text and Comments on Kaguru Notions of Sexuality," *Cahiers d'Études Africaines* 12, no. 45 (1972); Jean-Francois Bayart, *The State in Africa: The Politics of the Belly* (London: Longman, 1993); Mbembe, *On the Postcolony.*

36. Julia Kristeva, *Powers of Horror: An Essay on Abjection* (New York: Columbia University Press, 1982), 4.

37. Birgit Meyer, "'Praise the Lord': Popular Cinema and Pentecostalite Style in Ghana's New Public Sphere," *American Ethnologist* 31, no. 1 (2004): 92–110.

38. Asad, *Formations of the Secular,* 157.

39. See Harri Englund, *Prisoners of Freedom: Human Rights and the African Poor* (Berkeley: University of California Press, 2006).

40. Laidlaw, "For an Anthropology of Ethics and Freedom."

41. Karlström, "Modernity and Its Aspirants."

42. Wyrod, "Between Women's Rights and Men's Authority."

Epilogue

1. The concept of "disease across boundries" refers to Sandra Teresa Hyde, *Eating Spring Rice: The Cultural Politics of AIDS in Southwestern China* (Berkeley: University of California Press, 2007), 3.

2. Johanna Tayloe Crane, *Scrambling for Africa: AIDS, Expertise, and the Rise of American Global Health Science* (Ithaca, NY: Cornell University Press, 2013), 7.

BIBLIOGRAPHY

Archives in Uganda

Church of Uganda Provincial Archives, Uganda Christian University, Mukono, Uganda.
Bishop's Papers (Bp).
    Bp 178.1004. "Marriage of Natives in Uganda 1931, 1937."
    Bp 178.1005. "Marriage of Natives in Uganda 1938."
    Bp 178.1006. "Marriage of Natives in Uganda 1931."
    Bp 179.1012. "Marriage, Relationships, 1945, 1946."

Published Sources

Abu-Lughod, Lila. *Veiled Sentiments: Honor and Poetry in a Bedouin Society.* Berkeley: University of California Press, 1986.
Ahearn, Laura M. *Invitations to Love: Literacy, Love Letters, and Social Change in Nepal.* Ann Arbor: University of Michigan Press, 2001.
Anderson, Allan. "Exorcism and Conversion to African Pentecostalism." *Exchange* 35, no. 1 (2006): 116–33.
Archambault, Edith, and Judith Boumendil. "Dilemmas of Public/Private Partnership in France." In *Dilemmas of the Welfare Mix: The New Structure of Welfare in an Age of Privatization,* edited by Ugo Ascoli and Costanzo Ranci, 109–34. New York: Springer, 2002.
Asad, Talal. *Formations of the Secular: Christianity, Islam, Modernity.* Stanford, CA: Stanford University Press, 2003.
Ashforth, Adam. *Witchcraft, Violence, and Democracy in South Africa.* Chicago: University Chicago Press, 2005.
Barker, John. "Introduction." In *The Anthropology of Morality in Melanesia and Beyond,* edited by John Barker and Pamela J. Stewart, 1–21. New York: Ashgate, 2007.
Barnes, Sandra. *Patrons and Power: Creating a Political Community in Contemporary Lagos.* Manchester, England: Manchester University Press, 1986.
Bayart, Jean-Francois. *The State in Africa: The Politics of the Belly.* London: Longman, 1993.
Behrend, Heike. *Alice Lakwena and Holy Spirits: War in Northern Uganda, 1986–97.* Athens: Ohio University Press, 2000.
———. "The Rise of Occult Powers: AIDS and the Roman Catholic Church in Western Uganda." *Journal of Religion in Africa* 37, no. 1 (2007): 41–58.
Beidelman, T. O. *The Cool Knife: Imagery of Gender, Sexuality and Moral Education in Kaguru Initiation.* Washington, DC: Smithsonian Institution Press, 1997.
———. "The Filth of Incest: A Text and Comments on Kaguru Notions of Sexuality." *Cahiers d'Études Africaines* 12, no. 45 (1972): 164–73.

————. *Moral Imagination in Kaguru Modes of Thought.* Washington, DC: Smithsonian Institution Press, 1986.

Bialecki, John, Naomi Haynes, and Joel Robbins. "The Anthropology of Christianity." *Religion Compass* 2, no. 6 (2008): 1139–58.

Bledsoe, Caroline. *Women and Marriage in Kpelle Society.* Stanford, CA: Stanford University Press, 1980.

Boellstorff, Tom. "Between Religion and Desire: Being Muslim and *Gay* in Indonesia." *American Anthropologist* 107, no. 4 (2005): 575–85.

————. "Queer Studies in the House of Anthropology." *Annual Review of Anthropology* 36 (2007): 17–25.

Booth, Karen. *Local Women, Global Science: Fighting AIDS in Kenya.* Bloomington: Indiana University Press, 2004.

Bornstein, Erica. *Disquieting Gifts: Humanitarianism in New Delhi.* Stanford, CA: Stanford University Press, 2012.

Bornstein, Erica, and Peter Redfield. *Forces of Compassion: Humanitarianism between Ethics and Politics.* Santa Fe, NM: SAR, 2010.

Bourgois, Phillip. "The Moral Economies of Homeless Heroin Addicts: Confronting Ethnography, HIV Risk, and Everyday Violence in San Francisco Shooting Encampments." *Substance Use and Misuse* 33, no. 11 (1998): 2323–51.

Boyd, Lydia. "The Problem with Freedom: Homosexuality and Human Rights in Uganda." *Anthropological Quarterly* 86, no. 3 (2013): 697–724.

Brier, Jennifer. *Infectious Ideas: U.S. Political Responses to the AIDS Crisis.* Chapel Hill: University of North Carolina Press, 2011.

Brown, Peter. *The Body and Society: Men, Women, and Sexual Renunciation in Early Christianity.* Twentieth anniversary ed. New York: Columbia University Press, 2008.

Brusco, Elizabeth. *The Reformation of Machismo: Evangelical Conversion and Gender in Colombia.* Austin: University of Texas Press, 1995.

Burkhalter, Holly. "The Politics of AIDS: Engaging Conservative Activists." *Foreign Affairs* 83, no. 8 (2004): 8–14.

Burrill, Emily. *States of Marriage: Gender, Justice, and Rights in Colonial Mali.* Athens: Ohio University Press, 2015.

Caldwell, John, Pat Caldwell, and Pat Quiggin. "The Social Context of AIDS in Sub-Saharan Africa." *Population and Development Review* 15, no. 2 (1989): 185–234.

Campbell, Catherine. *Letting Them Die: Why HIV Prevention Programs Fail.* Oxford: Currey, 2003.

Cannell, Fenella. "The Christianity of Anthropology." In *The Anthropology of Christianity*, edited by Fenella Cannell, 1–50. Durham, NC: Duke University Press, 2005.

Cohen, Jonathan, and Tony Tate. "The Less They Know the Better: Abstinence-Only HIV Programs in Uganda." *Reproductive Health Matters* 14, no. 28 (2006): 174–78.

Cohen, Susan. "Beyond Slogans: Lessons from Uganda's Experience with ABC and HIV/AIDS." *Reproductive Health Matters* 12, no. 23 (2004): 132–35.

Cole, Jennifer. "Fresh Contact in Tamatave, Madagascar." *American Ethnologist* 31, no. 4 (2004): 573–88.

———. *Sex and Salvation: Imagining the Future in Madagascar.* Chicago: University of Chicago Press, 2010.

Coleman, Simon. *The Globalisation of Charismatic Christianity: Spreading the Gospel of Prosperity.* Cambridge: Cambridge University Press, 2000.

Comaroff, Jean. *Body of Power, Spirit of Resistance: The Culture and History of a South African People.* Chicago: University of Chicago Press, 1985.

———. "Healing and the Cultural Order: The Case of the Barolong boo Ratshidi." *American Ethnologist* 7, no. 4 (1980): 637–57.

Comaroff, Jean, and John L. Comaroff. "Millennial Capitalism and the Culture of Neoliberalism." *Public Culture* 12, no. 2 (2000): 291–343.

———. *Of Revelation and Revolution.* Vol. 1, *Christianity, Colonialism, and Consciousness in South Africa.* Chicago: University of Chicago Press, 1997.

Comaroff, John L., and Jean Comaroff. *Of Revelation and Revolution.* Vol. 2, *The Dialectics of Modernity on a South African Frontier.* Chicago: University of Chicago Press, 1997.

Copson, Raymond W. "AIDS in Africa." In *AIDS in Africa: A Pandemic on the Move*, edited by Garson Claton, 1–25. Hauppauge, NY: Nova Science, 2006.

Cornwall, Andrea, Sonia Corrêa, and Susie Jolly, eds. *Development with a Body: Sexuality, Human Rights and Development.* New York: Zed, 2008.

Corten, Andre, and Ruth Marshall-Fratani, eds. *Between Babel and Pentecost: Transnational Pentecostalism in Africa and Latin America.* London: Hurst, 2001.

Cowan, Jane K. "Culture and Rights after *Culture and Rights.*" *American Anthropologist* 108, no. 1 (2006): 9–24.

Crane, Johanna Tayloe. *Scrambling for Africa: AIDS, Expertise, and the Rise of American Global Health Science.* Ithaca, NY: Cornell University Press, 2013.

Cruikshank, Barbara. *The Will to Empower: Democratic Citizens and Other Subjects.* Ithaca, NY: Cornell University Press, 1999.

Csordas, Thomas J. *The Sacred Self: A Cultural Phenomenology of Charismatic Healing.* Berkeley: University of California Press, 1997.

Dabhoiwala, Faramerz. *The Origins of Sex: A History of the First Sexual Revolution.* Oxford: Oxford University Press, 2012.

Das, Pam. "Is Abstinence-Only Threatening Uganda's HIV Success Story?" *Lancet Infectious Diseases* 5, no. 5 (2005): 263–64.

Davis, Paula Jean. "On the Sexuality of 'Town Women' in Kampala." *Africa Today* 47, no. 3 (2000): 28–61.

Deeb, Laura. *An Enchanted Modern: Gender and Public Piety in Lebanon.* Princeton, NJ: Princeton University Press, 2006.

Dietrich, John W. "The Politics of PEPFAR: The President's Emergency Plan for AIDS Relief." *Ethics and International Affairs* 21, no. 3 (2007): 277–92.

Dilger, Hansorg. " 'We Are All Going to Die': Kinship, Belonging, and the Morality of HIV/AIDS-Related Illnesses and Deaths in Rural Tanzania." *Anthropological Quarterly* 81, no. 1 (2008): 207–32.

Donham, Donald L. "Freeing South Africa: The 'Modernization' of Male-Male Sexuality in Soweto." *Cultural Anthropology* 13, no. 1 (1998): 3–21.

Doyle, Shane. "Premarital Sexuality in Great Lakes Africa, 1900–1980." In *Generations Past: Youth in East African History*, edited by Andrew Burton and Helene Charton-Bigot, 237–61. Athens: Ohio University Press, 2010.

Duff, Oliver. "Public Health and Religion: AIDS, America, Abstinence." *Independent* (United Kingdom), June 1, 2006.

Dumont, Louis. "A Modified View of Our Origins: The Christian Beginnings of Modern Individualism." *Religion* 12, no. 1 (1982): 1–27.

Elisha, Omri. *Moral Ambition: Mobilization and Social Outreach in Evangelical Megachurches*. Berkeley: University of California Press, 2011.

Engelke, Matthew. *The Problem of Presence: Beyond Scripture in an African Church*. Berkeley: University of California Press, 2007.

———. "'We Wondered What Human Rights He Was Talking About': Human Rights, Homosexuality and the Zimbabwean Book Fair." *Critique of Anthropology* 19, no. 3 (1999): 289–314.

Engels, Friedrich. *Origin of the Family, Private Property, and the State*. Harmondsworth, England: Penguin, 1985.

Englund, Harri. *Prisoners of Freedom: Human Rights and the African Poor*. Berkeley: University of California Press, 2006.

Epprecht, Mark. *Heterosexual Africa? The History of an Idea from the Age of Exploration to the Age of AIDS*. Athens: Ohio University Press, 2008.

———. *Hungochani: The History of a Dissident Sexuality in Southern Africa*. Toronto: McGill-Queen's University Press, 2004.

———. "The Unsaying of Indigenous Homosexualities in Zimbabwe: Mapping a Blindspot in an African Masculinity." *Journal of Southern African Studies* 24, no. 4 (1998): 631–51.

Epstein, Helen. "God and the Fight against AIDS." *New York Review of Books* 52, no. 7 (2005): 47–49.

———. *The Invisible Cure: Africa, the West, and the Fight against AIDS*. New York: Farrar, Straus and Giroux, 2007.

Evans, Catrin, and Helen Lambert. "Implementing Community Interventions for HIV Prevention: Insights from Project Ethnography." *Social Science and Medicine* 66, no. 2 (2008): 467–78.

Evans-Pritchard, E. E. *Witchcraft, Oracles and Magic among the Azande*. Oxford: Oxford University Press, 1976.

Fassin, Didier. *Humanitarian Reason: A Moral History of the Present*. Berkeley: University of California Press, 2012.

Feierman, Stephen. *Health and Society in Africa: A Working Bibliography*. Honolulu, HI: Crossroads Press, 1979.

———. "Struggles for Control: The Social Basis of Health and Healing in Africa." *African Studies Review* 28, nos. 2–3 (1985): 73–147.

Feierman, Stephen, and John Janzen. *The Social Basis of Healing in Africa*. Berkeley: University of California Press, 1992.

Ferguson, James. *The Anti-Politics Machine: Development, Depoliticization, and Bureaucratic Power in Lesotho.* Minneapolis: University of Minnesota Press, 1994.

———. "The Uses of Neoliberalism." *Antipode* 41, no. s1 (2010): 166–84.

Finnström, Sverker. *Living with Bad Surroundings: War, History, and Everyday Moments in Northern Uganda.* Durham, NC: Duke University Press, 2008.

Foucault, Michel. *The Birth of Biopolitics: Lectures at the College de France, 1978–1979.* Translated by Graham Burchell. New York: Palgrave Macmillan, 2008.

———. *The History of Sexuality.* Vol. 1, *An Introduction.* Translated by Robert Hurley. New York: Vintage, 1978.

———. "Technologies of the Self." In *Technologies of the Self: A Seminar with Michel Foucault,* edited by Luther H. Martin, Huck Gutman, and Patrick H. Hutton, 16–49. Amherst: University of Massachusetts Press, 1988.

Gamson, Josh. "Silence, Death and the Invisible Enemy: AIDS Activism and Social Movement 'Newness.'" *Social Problems* 36, no. 4 (1989): 351–67.

Gardner, Christine J. *Making Chastity Sexy: The Rhetoric of Evangelical Abstinence Campaigns.* Chicago: University of Chicago Press, 2011.

Geertz, Clifford. "Thick Description: Toward an Interpretive Theory of Culture." In *The Interpretation of Cultures,* 3–32. New York: Basic Books, 1973.

Geisler, Wenzel, and Felicitas Becker, eds. *AIDS and Religious Practice in Africa.* Boston: Brill, 2009.

Geschiere, Peter. *The Modernity of Witchcraft: Politics and the Occult in Postcolonial Africa.* Charlottesville: University of Virginia Press, 1997.

Gill, Lesley. "'Like a Veil to Cover Them': Women and the Pentecostal Movement in La Paz." *American Ethnologist* 17, no. 4 (1990): 709–21.

Ginsburg, Faye. *Contested Lives: The Abortion Debate in an American Community.* Berkeley: University of California Press, 1986.

Ginsburg, Faye, and Rayna Rapp, eds. *Conceiving the New World Order: The Global Politics of Reproduction.* Berkeley: University of California Press, 1995.

Goetz, Anne Marie. "No Shortcuts to Power: Constraints on Women's Political Effectiveness in Uganda." *Journal of Modern African Studies* 40, no. 4 (2002): 549–75.

Goheen, Miriam. *Men Own the Fields, Women Own the Crops: Gender and Power in the Cameroon Grasslands.* Madison: University of Wisconsin Press, 1996.

Goldstein, Donna. "Microenterprise Training Programs, Neoliberal Common Sense, and the Discourses of Self-Esteem." In *The New Poverty Studies: The Ethnography of Power, Politics, and Impoverished People in the United States,* edited by Judith Goode and Jeff Maskovsky, 236–72. New York: New York University Press, 2001.

Good, Byron J. *Medicine, Rationality and Experience: An Anthropological Perspective.* Cambridge: Cambridge University Press, 1994.

Government Accountability Office. "Fighting AIDS in Uganda: What Went Right?" Hearing before the Senate Subcommittee on African Affairs, 108th Cong., 1st Session, S. Hrg. 108-106, May 19, 2003. Washington, DC: U.S. Government Printing Office.

———. "HIV/AIDS, TB, and Malaria: Combating a Global Pandemic." Hearing before the House Subcommittee on Health, 108th Cong., 1st Session, Serial no. 108-10, March 20, 2003. Washington, DC: U.S. Government Printing Office.

Government of Uganda. *UNGASS Country Progress Report Uganda January 2006 to December 2007*. Geneva: World Health Organization, 2008. http://library.health.go.ug/publications/service-delivery-diseases-control-prevention-commu nicable-diseases/hivaids/ungass.

Green, Edward C. *Rethinking AIDS Prevention: Learning from Successes in Developing Countries*. New York: Praeger, 2003.

Green, Edward C., Daniel T. Halperin, Vinand Nantulya, and Janice A. Hogle. "Uganda's HIV Prevention Success: The Role of Sexual Behavior Change and the National Response." *AIDS and Behavior* 10, no. 4 (2006): 335–46.

Green, Edward C., and Allison Herling Ruark. *AIDS Behavior and Culture: Understanding Evidence-Based Prevention*. Walnut Creek, CA: Left Coast, 2011.

Gupta, Geeta Rao, Justin Parkhurst, Jessica Ogden, Peter Aggleton, and Ajay Mahal. "Structural Approaches to HIV Prevention." *Lancet* 372, no. 9640 (2008): 764–75.

Gussman, Alessandro. "HIV/AIDS, Pentecostal Churches, and the Joseph Generation in Uganda." *Africa Today* 56, no. 1 (2009): 67–86.

Guyer, Jane. "Wealth in People and Self-Realization in Equatorial Africa." *Man* 28, no. 2 (1993): 243–65.

Guyer, Jane, and Samuel Belinga. "Wealth in People as Wealth in Knowledge: Accumulation and Composition in Equatorial Africa." *Journal of African History* 36, no. 1 (1995): 91–120.

Hamdy, Sherine. *Our Bodies Belong to God: Organ Transplants, Islam, and the Struggle for Human Dignity in Egypt*. Berkeley: University of California Press, 2012.

Hansen, Holger Bernt. *Mission, Church, and State in a Colonial Setting: Uganda, 1890–1925*. New York: St. Martin's, 1984.

Hanson, Holly. *Landed Obligation: The Practice of Power in Buganda*. Portsmouth, NH: Heinemann, 2003.

Harding, Susan. *The Book of Jerry Falwell: Fundamentalist Language and Politics*. Princeton, NJ: Princeton University Press, 2001.

———. "Representing Fundamentalism: The Problem of the Repugnant Cultural Other." *Social Research* 58, no. 2 (1991): 373–93.

Harvey, David. *A Brief History of Neoliberalism*. Oxford: Oxford University Press, 2005.

———. *The Condition of Postmodernity*. New York: Blackwell, 1989.

Heald, Suzette. *Manhood and Morality: Sex, Violence and Ritual in Gisu Society*. New York: Routledge, 1999.

———. "The Power of Sex: Some Reflections of the Caldwells' 'African Sexuality' Thesis." *Africa* 65, no. 4 (1995): 489–505.

Heise, Lori L., and Christopher Elias. "Transforming AIDS Prevention to Meet Women's Needs: A Focus on Developing Countries." *Social Science and Medicine* 40, no. 7 (1995): 931–43.

Hirschkind, Charles. *The Ethical Soundscape: Cassette Sermons and Islamic Counterpublics*. New York: Columbia University Press, 2006.

Hoad, Neville. *African Intimacies: Race, Homosexuality, and Globalization*. Minneapolis: University of Minnesota Press, 2007.

Hofer, Katharina. "The Role of Evangelical NGOs in International Development: A Comparative Case Study of Kenya and Uganda." *Africa Spectrum* 38, no. 3 (2003): 375–98.

Human Rights Watch. "The Less They Know, the Better: Abstinence-Only HIV/AIDS Programs in Uganda." http://hrw.org/reports/2005/uganda0305/.

Hunt, Nancy. *A Colonial Lexicon: Of Birth Ritual, Medicalization, and Mobility in the Congo*. Durham, NC: Duke University Press, 1999.

———. "Condoms, Confessors, Conferences: Among AIDS Derivatives in Africa." *Journal of the International Institute* 4, no. 3 (1997): 15–17.

Hunt, Stephen. "'Neither Here nor There': The Construction of Identities and Boundary Maintenance of West African Pentecostals." *Sociology* 36, no. 1 (2002): 146–69.

Hunter, Mark. "Cultural Politics and Masculinities: Multiple-Partners in Historical Perspective in KwaZulu-Natal." *Culture, Health and Sexuality* 7, no. 4 (2005): 389–403.

———. *Love in the Time of AIDS*. Bloomington: Indiana University Press, 2010.

Hutchinson, Sharon. "The Cattle of Money and the Cattle of Girls among the Nuer, 1930–83." *American Ethnologist* 19, no. 2 (1992): 294–316.

Hyde, Sandra Teresa. *Eating Spring Rice: The Cultural Politics of AIDS in Southwestern China*. Berkeley: University of California Press, 2007.

Iliffe, John. *The African AIDS Epidemic: A History*. Oxford: Currey, 2006.

———. *Honour in African History*. Cambridge: Cambridge University Press, 2005.

"Is It Churlish to Criticise Bush over His Spending on AIDS?" *Lancet* 364, no. 9431 (2004): 303–4.

Iyamuremye, Betty. "Marriage and Divorce Bill to Protect Marriages." *New Vision* (Uganda), March 19, 2013. http://www.newvision.co.ug/news/640829-marriage-and-divorce-bill-to-protect-marriages.html.

James, Erica Caple. *Democratic Insecurities: Violence, Trauma, and Intervention in Haiti*. Berkeley: University of California Press, 2010.

Jeannerat, Caroline. "Of Lizards, Misfortune and Deliverance: Pentecostal Soteriology in the Life of a Migrant." *African Studies* 68, no. 2 (2009): 251–71.

Jenkins, Philip. *The Next Christendom: The Coming of Global Christianity*. Oxford: Oxford University Press, 2002.

Jones, Ben. *Beyond the State in Rural Uganda*. Edinburgh: Edinburgh University Press, 2009.

Kagwa, Apolo. *The Customs of the Baganda*. Translated by Ernest B. Kalibala. New York: Columbia University Press, 1934.

———. *The Kings of Buganda*. Translated by M. S. M. Kiwanuka. Nairobi, Kenya: East African Publishing House, 1971.

Kaler, Amy. *Running After Pills*. Portsmouth, NH: Heinemann, 2003.

Karlström, Mikael. "Imagining Democracy: Political Culture and Democratisation in Buganda." *Africa* 66, no. 4 (1996): 485–505.

———. "Modernity and Its Aspirants: Moral Community and Development Eutopianism in Buganda." *Current Anthropology* 45, no. 4 (2004): 595–610.

Kasfir, Nelson. "Guerrillas and Civilian Participation: The National Resistance Army in Uganda, 1981–86." *Journal of Modern African Studies* 43, no. 2 (2005): 271–96.

Kasule, Samuel. "Popular Performance and the Construction of Social Reality in Post-Amin Uganda." *Journal of Popular Culture* 32, no. 2 (1998): 39–58.

Keane, Webb. *Christian Moderns: Freedom and Fetish in the Mission Encounter.* Berkeley: University of California Press, 2007.

———. "Sincerity, 'Modernity,' and the Protestants." *Cultural Anthropology* 17, no. 1 (2002): 65–92.

Kinsman, John. *AIDS Policy in Uganda: Evidence, Ideology, and the Making of an African Success Story.* New York: Palgrave Macmillan, 2010.

Kirby, Douglas, and David Halperin. "Success in Uganda: An Analysis of Behavior Change that Led to Declines in HIV Prevalence in the Early 1990s." ETR Associates, Santa Cruz, CA, 2008.

Kiwanuka, M. S. M. *A History of Buganda: From the Foundation of the Kingdom to 1900.* London: Longman, 1971.

Kiwuuwa, Paul. "Homosexual Admits Recruiting Students." *New Vision* (Uganda), March 23, 2009. http://www.newvision.co.ug/PA/8/12/675619.

Klaits, Frederick. *Death in a Church of Life: Moral Passion during Botswana's Time of AIDS.* Berkeley: University of California Press, 2010.

Kleinman, Arthur. *Living a Moral Life amidst Uncertainty and Danger.* Oxford: Oxford University Press, 2007.

Kodesh, Neil. *Beyond the Royal Gaze: Clanship and Public Healing in Uganda.* Charlottesville: University of Virginia Press, 2010.

Kristeva, Julia. *Powers of Horror: An Essay on Abjection.* New York: Columbia University Press, 1982.

Kron, Josh. "Resentment towards West Bolsters Uganda's New Anti-Gay Bill." *New York Times,* February 28, 2012.

Kuypers, Jim A., Megan Hitchner, James Irwin, and Alexander Wilson. "Compassionate Conservatism: The Rhetorical Reconstruction of Conservative Rhetoric." *American Communication Journal* 6, no. 4 (2003): 1–27.

Kyomuhendo, Grace Bantebya, and Marjorie Keniston McIntosh. *Women, Work and Domestic Virtue in Uganda (1900–2003).* Oxford: Currey, 2006.

Laidlaw, James. "For an Anthropology of Ethics and Freedom." *Journal of the Royal Anthropological Institute* 8, no. 2 (2002): 311–32.

Langwick, Stacey. *Bodies, Politics and African Healing: The Matter of Maladies in Tanzania.* Bloomington: Indiana University Press, 2011.

Lehmann, David. *Struggle for the Spirit: Religious Transformation and Popular Culture in Brazil and Latin America.* Cambridge: Blackwell, 1996.

Li, Tania. *The Will to Improve: Governmentality, Development, and the Practice of Politics.* Durham, NC: Duke University Press, 2007.

Lienhardt, Godfrey. "Self: Public and Private—Some African Representations." In *The Category of the Person: Anthropology, Philosophy, History,* edited by Michael

Carrithers, Steven Collins, and Steven Lukes, 141–55. Cambridge: Cambridge University Press, 1985.

Lindhardt, Martin. "The Ambivalence of Power: Charismatic Christianity and Occult Forces in Urban Tanzania." *Nordic Journal of Religion and Society* 22, no. 1 (2009): 37–54.

LiPuma, Edward. "Modernity and Forms of Personhood in Melanesia." In *Bodies and Persons: Comparative Perspectives from Africa and Melanesia*, edited by Michael Lambek and Andrew Strathern, 53–79. Cambridge: Cambridge University Press, 1998.

Livingston, Julie. *Debility and the Moral Imagination in Botswana*. Bloomington: Indiana University Press, 2005.

Low, D. A. *Buganda in Modern History*. Berkeley: University of California Press, 1971.

Low-Beer, Daniel, and Rand L. Stoneburner. "Behaviour and Communication Change in Reducing HIV: Is Uganda Unique?" *African Journal of AIDS Research* 2, no. 1 (2003): 9–21.

Lowenstein, George F., Elke Webber, Christopher Hsee, and Ned Welsh. "Risk as Feelings." *Psychological Bulletin* 127, no. 2 (2001): 267–86.

Lutz, Catherine A. *Unnatural Emotions: Everyday Sentiments on a Micronesian Atoll and Their Challenge to Western Theory*. Chicago: University of Chicago Press, 1988.

Lyon, David. *Jesus in Disneyland: Religion in Postmodern Times*. Cambridge: Polity, 2000.

Lyons, Maryinez. "Mobile Populations and HIV/AIDS in East Africa." In *HIV and AIDS in Africa: Beyond Epidemiology*, edited by Ezekiel Kalipeni, Susan Craddock, Joseph R. Oppong, and Jayati Gosh, 175–90. Malden, MA: Blackwell, 2004.

Mah, Timothy L., and Daniel Halperin. "Concurrent Sexual Partnerships and the HIV Epidemic in Africa: Evidence to Move Forward." *AIDS and Behavior* 14, no. 1 (2010): 11–16.

Mahmood, Saba. *Politics of Piety: The Islamic Revival and the Feminist Subject*. Princeton, NJ: Princeton University Press, 2005.

Mains, Daniel. "Blackouts and Progress: Privatization, Infrastructure, and the Developmentalist State in Jimma, Ethiopia." *Cultural Anthropology* 27, no. 1 (2012): 3–27.

Mair, Lucy. *African Marriage and Social Change*. London: Cass, 1969.

———. *An African People in the Twentieth Century*. New York: Russell and Russell, 1934.

———. *Native Marriage in Buganda*. International Institute of African Languages and Cultures Memorandum 19. London: Oxford University Press, 1940.

Malinowski, Bronislaw. *Argonauts of the Western Pacific*. Prospect Heights, IL: Waveland, 1984.

Mamdani, Mahmood. *Scholars in the Marketplace: The Dilemmas of Neo-liberal Reform at Makerere University, 1989–2005*. Dakar, Senegal: CODESRIA, 2007.

Marshall, Ruth. *Political Spiritualities: The Pentecostal Revolution in Nigeria*. Chicago: University of Chicago Press, 2009.

Martin, David. *On Secularisation*. London: Ashgate, 2005.

————. *Pentecostalism: The World Their Parish.* Oxford: Blackwell, 2002.

Martin, Emily. *Flexible Bodies: The Role of Immunity in American Culture from the Days of Polio to the Age of AIDS.* Boston: Beacon, 1994.

Mauss, Marcel. *The Gift: The Form and Reason for Exchange in Archaic Societies.* New York: Norton, 2000.

Mbembe, Achille. "African Modes of Self-Writing." *Public Culture* 14, no. 1 (2003): 239–73.

————. *On the Postcolony.* Berkeley: University of California Press, 2001.

Mbiti, John. *African Religions and Philosophy.* London: Heinemann, 1992.

Merry, Sally Engel. "Transnational Human Rights and Local Activism." *American Anthropologist* 108, no. 1 (2006): 38–51.

Meyer, Birgit. "'Make a Complete Break with the Past': Memory and Postcolonial Modernity in Ghanaian Pentecostal Discourse." *Journal of Religion in Africa* 28, no. 3 (1998): 316–49.

————. "'Praise the Lord': Popular Cinema and Pentecostalite Style in Ghana's New Public Sphere." *American Ethnologist* 31, no. 1 (2004): 92–110.

————. *Translating the Devil: Religion and Modernity among the Ewe of Ghana.* Trenton, NJ: Africa World Press, 1999.

Meyer, Birgit, and Peter Pels, eds. *Magic and Modernity: Interfaces of Revelation and Concealment.* Stanford, CA: Stanford University Press, 2003.

Miers, Susan, and Igor Koytoff, eds. *Slavery in Africa: Historical and Anthropological Perspectives.* Madison: University of Wisconsin Press, 1977.

Mills, David, and Richard Ssewakiryanga. "'No Romance without Finance': Masculinities, Commodities and HIV in Uganda." In *Readings in Gender in Africa*, edited by Andrea Cornwall, 90–94. Oxford: Currey, 2005.

Mirembe, Robinah. "AIDS and Democratic Education in Uganda." *Comparative Education* 38, no. 3 (2002): 291–302.

Moore, Henrietta L., and Todd Sanders, eds. *Magical Interpretations, Material Realities: Modernity, Witchcraft and the Occult in Postcolonial Africa.* London: Routledge, 2001.

Morgan, Sandra, and Jeff Maskovsky. "The Anthropology of Welfare 'Reform': New Perspectives on U.S. Urban Poverty in the Post-Welfare Era." *Annual Review of Anthropology* 32 (2003): 315–38.

Muehlebach, Andrea. *The Moral Neoliberal: Welfare and Citizenship in Italy.* Chicago: University of Chicago Press, 2012.

Mukama, Ruth. "Women's Discourses as the Conservators of Cultural Values in Language." *International Journal of the Sociology of Language* 129, no. 1 (1998): 157–66.

Murphy, Elaine, Margaret Greene, Alexandra Mihailovic, and Peter Olupot-Olupot. "Was the ABC Approach (Abstinence, Being Faithful, Using Condoms) Responsible for Uganda's Decline in HIV?" *PLoS Medicine* 3, no. 9 (2006): e379.

Museveni, Yoweri. *Sowing the Mustard Seed: The Struggle for Freedom and Democracy in Uganda.* New York: Macmillan Educational, 1997.

————. *What Is Africa's Problem?* Minneapolis: University of Minnesota Press, 1992.

Musisi, Nakanyike B. "Gender and the Cultural Construction of 'Bad Women' in the Development of Kampala-Kibuga, 1900–1962." *In "Wicked" Women and the Reconfiguration of Gender in Africa*, edited by Dorothy L. Hodgson and Sheryl A. McCurdy, 171–87. Portsmouth, NH: Heinemann, 2001.

———. "Morality as Identity: the Missionary Moral Agenda in Buganda, 1877–1945." *Journal of Religious History* 23, no. 1 (1999): 51–74.

———. "Women, 'Elite Polygyny,' and Buganda State Formation." *Signs* 16, no. 4 (1991): 757–86.

Mutumba, Haji Nsereko. "Loopholes in the Marriage and Divorce Bill." *New Vision* (Uganda), April, 2, 2013. http://www.newvision.co.ug/news/641265-loopholes -in-the-marriage-and-divorce-bill.html.

Mwenda, Andrew. "Uganda's Politics of Foreign Aid and Violent Conflict: The Political Uses of the LRA Rebellion." In *The Lord's Resistance Army: Myth and Reality*, edited by Tim Allen and Koen Vlassenroot, 45–54. London: Zed, 2010.

Nguyen, Vinh-Kim. *The Republic of Therapy: Triage and Sovereignty in West Africa's Time of AIDS*. Durham, NC: Duke University Press, 2010.

Niehaus, Isak. "Perversion of Power: Witchcraft and the Sexuality of Evil in the South African Lowveld." *Journal of Religion in Africa* 32, no. 3 (2002): 269–99.

Nyanzi, Barbara, Stella Nyanzi, Brent Wolff, and James Whitworth. "Money, Men and Markets: Economic and Sexual Empowerment of Market Women in Southwestern Uganda." *Culture, Health and Sexuality* 7, no. 1 (2006): 13–26.

Obbo, Christine. "Dominant Male Ideology and Female Options: Three African Case Studies." *Africa* 46, no. 4 (1976): 371–89.

Ogden, Jessica A. "'Producing' Respect: The 'Proper Woman' in Postcolonial Kampala." In *Postcolonial Identities in Africa*, edited by R. P. Werbner and T. O. Ranger, 165–92. New York: Zed, 1996.

Ong, Aihwa. *Neoliberalism as Exception: Mutations in Citizenship and Sovereignty*. Durham, NC: Duke University Press, 2006.

Osborn, Emily Lynn. *Our New Husbands Are Here: Households, Gender and Politics in a West African State from the Slave Trade to Colonial Rule*. Athens: Ohio University Press, 2011.

Paley, Julia. *Marketing Democracy: Power and Social Movements in Post-Dictatorship Peru*. Berkeley: University of California Press, 2001.

Parikh, Shanti. "'Don't Tell Your Sister or Anyone That You Love Me': Considering the Effects of Adult Regulation on Adolescent Sexual Subjectivities in Uganda's Time of AIDS." In *Gender, Sexuality and HIV/AIDS: Research and Intervention in Africa*, edited by Britt Pinkowsky Tersbøl, 53–84. Copenhagen: Institute of Public Health, University of Copenhagen, 2003.

———. "From Auntie to Disco: The Bifurcation of Risk and Pleasure in Sex Education in Uganda." In *Sex in Development: Science, Sexuality and Morality in Global Perspective*, edited by Vincanne Adams and Stacy Leigh Pigg, 125–58. Durham, NC: Duke University Press, 2005.

———. "The Political Economy of Marriage and HIV: The ABC Approach, 'Safe' Infidelity, and Managing Moral Risk in Uganda." *Framing Health Matters* 97, no. 7 (2007): 1198–1208.

———. "Sex, Lies and Love Letters: Condoms, Female Agency, and Paradoxes of Romance in Uganda." *Agenda: African Feminisms* 62, no. 1 (2004): 2–20.

———. "Sugar Daddies and Sexual Citizenship in Uganda: Rethinking Third Wave Feminism." *Black Renaissance / Renaissance Noir* 6, no. 1 (2004): 82–107.

———. "'They Arrested Me for Loving a Schoolgirl': Ethnography, HIV, and a Feminist Assessment of the Age of Consent Law as a Gender-Based Structural Intervention in Uganda." *Social Science and Medicine* 74, no. 11 (2012): 1774–82.

Parkhurst, Justin O. "Evidence, Politics and Uganda's HIV Success: Moving Forward with ABC and HIV Prevention." *Journal of International Development* 23, no. 2 (2011): 240–52.

Perez, Tina L., and George N. Dionisopoulos. "Presidential Silence, C. Everett Koop, and the Surgeon General's Report on AIDS." *Communication Studies* 46, nos. 1–2 (1995): 18–43.

Perrin, Karen, and Sharon Bernecki DeJoy. "Abstinence-Only Education: How We Got Here and Where We're Going." *Journal of Public Health Policy* 24, nos. 3–4 (2003): 445–59.

Petersen, Alan, and Deborah Lupton. *The New Public Health: Health and Self in the Age of Risk.* London: Sage, 1996.

Peterson, Derek R. *Ethnic Patriotism and the East African Revival: A History of Dissent, c. 1935–1972.* Cambridge: Cambridge University Press, 2012.

———. "Wordy Women: Gender Trouble and the Oral Politics of the East African Revival in Gikuyuland." *Journal of African History* 42, no. 3 (2001): 469–89.

Petryna, Adriana. "Experimentality: On the Global Mobility and Regulation of Human Subjects Research." *PoLAR* 30, no. 2 (2007): 288–304.

———. *Life Exposed: Biological Citizens after Chernobyl.* Princeton, NJ: Princeton University Press, 2003.

———. *When Experiments Travel: Clinical Trials and the Global Search for Human Subjects.* Princeton, NJ: Princeton University Press, 2009.

Pigg, Stacy Leigh, and Vincanne Adams. "Introduction: The Moral Object of Sex." In *Sex in Development: Science, Sexuality, and Morality in Global Perspective*, edited by Vincanne Adams and Stacy Leigh Pigg, 1–38. Durham, NC: Duke University Press, 2005.

Piot, Charles. *Nostalgia for the Future: West Africa after the Cold War.* Chicago: University of Chicago Press, 2010.

———. *Remotely Global: Village Modernity in West Africa.* Chicago: University of Chicago Press, 1999.

Posel, Deborah. "Afterword: Vigilantism and the Burden of Rights: Reflections on the Paradoxes of Freedom in Post-Apartheid South Africa." *African Studies* 63, no. 2 (2004): 231–36.

———. "The Scandal of Manhood: 'Baby Rape' and the Politicization of Sexual Violence in Post-Apartheid South Africa." *Culture, Health and Sexuality* 7, no. 3 (2005): 239–52.

Prince, Ruth. "HIV and the Moral Economy of Survival in an East African City." *Medical Anthropology Quarterly* 26, no. 4 (2012): 534–56.

Putzel, James. "The Politics of Action on AIDS: A Case Study of Uganda." *Public Administration and Development* 24, no. 1 (2004): 19–30.

Redfield, Peter. *Life in Crisis: The Ethical Journey of Doctors without Borders.* Berkeley: University of California Press, 2013.

Robbins, Joel. *Becoming Sinners: Christianity and Moral Torment in a Papua New Guinea Society.* Berkeley: University of California Press, 2004.

———. "The Globalization of Charismatic and Pentecostal Christianity." *Annual Review of Anthropology* 33 (2004): 117–43.

———. "On the Paradoxes of Global Pentecostalism and the Perils of Continuity Thinking." *Religion* 33, no. 3 (2003): 221–31.

Rödlach, Alexander. *Witches, Westerners, and HIV: AIDS and Cultures of Blame in Africa.* Walnut Creek, CA: Left Coast, 2006.

Rose, Nikolas. *The Politics of Life Itself.* Princeton, NJ: Princeton University Press, 2007.

———. *Powers of Freedom: Reframing Political Thought.* Cambridge: Cambridge University Press, 1999.

Rozin, Paul, and April E. Fallon. "A Perspective on Disgust." *Psychological Review* 94, no. 1 (1987): 23–41.

Rudnyckyj, Daromir. *Spiritual Economies: Islam, Globalization, and the Afterlife of Development.* Ithaca, NY: Cornell University Press, 2010.

Sadgrove, Jo. "'Keeping Up Appearances': Sex and Religion amongst University Students in Uganda." *Journal of Religion in Africa* 37, no. 1 (2007): 116–44.

Sadowsky, Jonathan. *Imperial Bedlam: Institutions of Madness in Colonial Southwest Nigeria.* Berkeley: University of California Press, 1999.

Scherz, China. *Having People, Having Heart: Charity, Sustainable Development, and the Problems of Dependence in Central Uganda.* Chicago: University of Chicago Press, 2014.

Schoepf, Brooke. "Museveni's Other War: Condoms in Uganda." *Review of African Political Economy* 31, no. 100 (2004): 372–76.

Seelye, Katherine Q. "Helms Puts the Brakes to a Bill Financing AIDS Treatment." *New York Times,* July 5, 1995. http://www.nytimes.com/1995/07/05/us/helms -puts-the-brakes-to-a-bill-financing-aids-treatment.html.

Sharlet, Jeff. *The Family: The Secret Fundamentalism at the Heart of American Power.* New York: HarperCollins, 2009.

———. "Straight Man's Burden: The American Roots of Uganda's Anti-Gay Persecution." *Harper's,* September 2010, 36–48.

Shaw, Rosalind. "'Tok Af, Lef Af': A Political Economy of Temne Techniques of Secrecy and Self." In *African Philosophy as Cultural Inquiry,* edited by Ivan Karp and D. A. Masolo, 25–49. Bloomington: Indiana University Press, 2000.

Shoaps, Robin. "'Pray Earnestly': The Textual Construction of Personal Involvement in Pentecostal Prayer and Song." *Journal of Linguistic Anthropology* 12, no. 1 (2002): 34–71.

Shore, Cris, and Susan Wright. *Anthropology of Policy: Perspectives on Governance and Power.* New York: Routledge, 1997.

Simmel, Georg. *The Philosophy of Money.* Translated by Tom Bottomore and David Frisby. London: Routledge, 1978.

———. "The Sociology of Secrecy and Secret Societies." Translated by Albion W. Small. *American Journal of Sociology* 11, no. 4 (1906): 441–98.

Simpson, Anthony. *Boys to Men in the Shadow of AIDS: Masculinities and HIV Risk in Zambia.* New York: Palgrave Macmillan, 2009.

Sinding, Steven W. "Does 'CNN' (Condoms, Needles and Negotiation) Work Better Than 'ABC' (Abstinence, Faithfulness and Condom Use) in Attacking the AIDS Epidemic?" *International Family Planning Perspectives* 31, no. 1 (2005): 38–40.

Smith, Daniel Jordan. *A Culture of Corruption: Everyday Deception and Popular Discontent in Nigeria.* Princeton, NJ: Princeton University Press, 2008.

———. "Romance, Parenthood, and Gender in a Modern African Society." *Ethnology* 40, no. 2 (2001): 129–51.

———. "Youth, Sin and Sex in Nigeria: Christianity and HIV/AIDS-Related Beliefs and Behaviour among Rural-Urban Migrants." *Culture, Health and Sexuality* 6, no. 5 (2004): 425–37.

Smith, James Howard. *Bewitching Development: Witchcraft and the Reinvention of Development in Neoliberal Kenya.* Chicago: University of Chicago Press, 2008.

Southall, A. W. and P. C. W. Gutkind. *Townsmen in the Making: Kampala and Its Suburbs.* Kampala, Uganda: East African Institute for Social Research, 1957.

Ssempa, Martin. "Homosexuality Is against Our Culture." *New Vision* (Uganda), September 5, 2007. Reprinted in *Homosexuality: Perspectives from Uganda,* edited by Sylvia Tamale, 41–44. Kampala, Uganda: Sexual Minorities of Uganda, 2007.

Ssempogo, Herbert. "Religious Groups Demonstrate against Homosexuals." *New Vision* (Uganda), August 21, 2007. http://www.newvision.co.ug/PA/8/12/582544.

Stewart, Kearsley. "Toward a Historical Perspective on Sexuality in Uganda: The Reproductive Lifeline Technique for Grandmothers and Their Daughters." *Africa Today* 47, nos. 3–4 (2001): 122–48.

Stokes, Wendy. *Women in Contemporary Politics.* Cambridge: Polity, 2005.

Stone, Lawrence. *The Family, Sex, and Marriage in England, 1500–1800.* New York: Harper and Row, 1977.

Stoneburner, Rand L., and Daniel Low-Beer. "Population-Level HIV Declines and Behavioral Risk Avoidance in Uganda." *Science* 304, no. 5671 (2004): 714–18.

Stroumsa, Guy G. "Caro salutis cardo: Shaping the Person in Early Christian Thought." *History of Religions* 30, no. 1 (1990): 25–50.

Sumartojo, Esther. "Structural Factors in HIV Prevention: Concepts, Examples, and Implications for Research." *AIDS* 14, suppl. 1 (2000): S3–10.

Summers, Carol. "Grandfathers, Grandsons, Morality, and Radical Politics in Late Colonial Buganda." *International Journal of African Historical Studies* 38, no. 3 (2005): 427–47.

Swezey, Teresa, and Michele Teitelbaum. "HIV/AIDS and the Context of Polygyny and Other Marital and Sexual Unions in Africa: Implications for Risk Assessment and Interventions." In *AIDS, Culture, and Africa,* edited by Douglas Feldman, 220–38. Gainesville: University of Florida Press, 2008.

Tamale, Sylvia. "Eroticism, Sensuality and 'Women's Secrets' among the Baganda: A Critical Analysis." *Feminist Africa* 5 (2005): 9–36.

———, ed. *Homosexuality: Perspectives from Uganda*. Kampala, Uganda: Sexual Minorities of Uganda, 2007.

———. "Out of the Closet: Unveiling Sexuality Discourses in Uganda." In *Africa after Gender?*, edited by Catherine M. Cole, Takyiwaa Manuh, and Stephan F. Miescher, 17–29. Bloomington: Indiana University Press, 2007.

———. *When Hens Begin to Crow: Gender and Parliamentary Politics in Uganda*. Boulder, CO: Westview Press, 1999.

Taylor, Charles. *The Sources of the Self: The Making of the Modern Identity*. Cambridge, MA: Harvard University Press, 1989.

Tempels, Placide. *Bantu Philosophy*. Paris: Presence Africaine, 1959.

Thomas, Lynn M., and Jennifer Cole. "Thinking through Love in Africa." In *Love in Africa*, edited by Jennifer Cole and Lynn M. Thomas, 1–30. Chicago: University of Chicago Press, 2009.

Thornton, Robert J. *Unimagined Community: Sex, Networks, and AIDS in Uganda and South Africa*. Berkeley: University of California Press, 2008.

Ticktin, Miriam. *Casualties of Care: Immigration and the Politics of Humanitarianism in France*. Berkeley: University of California Press, 2011.

Trilling, Lionel. *Sincerity and Authenticity*. Cambridge, MA: Harvard University Press, 1971.

Tsing, Anna. *In the Realm of the Diamond Queen: Marginality in an Out-of-the-Way Place*. Princeton, NJ: Princeton University Press, 1993.

Tumushabe, Joseph. *The Politics of HIV/AIDS in Uganda*. Geneva: United Nations Research Institute for Social Development, 2006.

Twaddle, Michael. *Kakungulu and the Creation of Uganda, 1868–1928*. London: Currey, 1993.

UNAIDS. *2004 Report on the Global AIDS Epidemic*. Geneva: UNAIDS, 2004.

U.S. Congress. House. Congressional Committee. *Rallying the Armies of Compassion*. 107th Cong., 1st Sess., 2001. H. Doc. 107–36.

United States President's Emergency Plan for AIDS Relief. *Fiscal Year 2005 Operational Plan, June 2005 Update*. Washington, DC: Office of the United States Global AIDS Coordinator, 2005.

———. *PEPFAR's Five-Year Strategy*. December 2009. http://www.pepfar.gov/about/strategy/document/133251.htm.

———. *Uganda Fiscal Year 2008 PEPFAR Country Operational Plan (COP)*. June 2008. http://www.pepfar.gov/about/opplan08/102010.htm.

Van Allen, Judith. "Sitting on a Man: Colonialism and the Lost Political Institutions of Igbo Women." *Canadian Journal of African Studies* 6, no. 2 (1972): 165–81.

Vaughan, Megan. *Curing Their Ills: Colonial Power and African Illness*. London: Polity, 1991.

Vincent, Louise. "Virginity Testing in South Africa: Re-traditioning the Postcolony." *Culture, Health and Sexuality* 8, no. 1 (2006): 17–30.

Wardlow, Holly, and Jennifer Hirsch. "Introduction." In *Modern Loves: The Anthropology of Romantic Courtship and Companionate Marriage*, edited by Holly

Wardlow and Jennifer Hirsch, 1–34. Ann Arbor: University of Michigan Press, 2006.

Weiner, Annette. *Inalienable Possessions*. Berkeley: University of California Press, 1992.

Weiss, Brad. *The Making and Unmaking of the Haya Lived World: Consumption, Commoditization, and Everyday Practice*. Durham, NC: Duke University Press, 1996.

Wendland, Claire L. *A Heart for the Work: Journeys through an African Medical School*. Chicago: University of Chicago Press, 2010.

West, Harry, and Todd Sanders, eds. *Transparency and Conspiracy: Ethnographies of Suspicion in the New World Order*. Durham, NC: Duke University Press, 2003.

White, Luise. *Speaking with Vampires: Rumor and History in Colonial Africa*. Berkeley: University of California Press, 2000.

Wilson, Richard Ashby, and Richard Brown. *Humanitarianism and Suffering: The Mobilization of Empathy*. Cambridge: Cambridge University Press, 2009.

Whyte, Susan Reynolds. *Questioning Misfortune: The Pragmatics of Uncertainty in Eastern Uganda*. Cambridge: Cambridge University Press, 1998.

Witte, Kim, and Mike Allen. "A Meta-Analysis of Fear Appeals: Implications for Effective Public Health Campaigns." *Health, Education and Behavior* 27, no. 5 (2000): 591–615.

Wrigley, C.C. "The Christian Revolution in Buganda." *Comparative Studies in Society and History* 2, no. 1 (1959): 33–58.

Wrigley, Christopher. *Kingship and State: The Buganda Dynasty*. Cambridge: Cambridge University Press, 1996.

Wyrod, Robert. "Between Women's Rights and Men's Authority: Masculinity and Discourses of Gender Difference in Urban Uganda." *Gender and Society* 22, no. 6 (2008): 799–823.

INDEX

relationships and, 122–26; structural inequalities and, 186. *See also* public health

Helms, Jesse, 27

Hirsch, Jennifer, 135

History of Sexuality (Foucault), 159

HIV/AIDS in Uganda: ABC prevention plan, 37, 40, 44–45, 47; born-again Christian activists and, 3–4, 16, 21–22, 29–30, 37–38, 50–53, *52*, 57, 71, 71–74, *131*; debates over, 1–2; drop in prevalence, 1–2, 42–44, 53, 185; funding, 35–36, 48; global response, 35–39; peer-to-peer education, 47, 50; policy making, 1–7; as state of crisis, 10–11, 14; treatment access, 36–37; Uganda civil war and, 55. *See also* abstinence and faithfulness programs; President's Emergency Plan for AIDS Relief (PEPFAR); public health

homosexuality: antihomosexuality movement, 17–18, 21–22, 157–58, 161, *162*, 162–64, 177–79, 183; fear of, 169–71; identity and, 159–60; as imported, 165; predatory, 168, 173; recruitment, 169–73, 172–74; secrecy and, 174–76; as spiritual threat, 173–76. *See also* Anti-Homosexuality Bill (Uganda); lesbianism

household and family: as political project, 57; reform of, 68–69, 73, 75; social change in Buganda, 58–63, 65–66; traditional, criticisms of, 97–102

humanitarianism, 4, 6–7, 8, 11, 12, 29, 34, 54, 185, 188n9. *See also* President's Emergency Plan for AIDS Relief (PEPFAR)

human rights: interpretations of, 166–67; neoliberalism and, 176–79

Human Rights Watch, 48

Iliffe, John, 91

incest, 168

individual accountability: access to services and, 6–7; American ideal of, 75–76, 80, 181; compassionate, 30–31, 34–35, 56; in neoliberalism, 8, 10, 11, 12, 14, 16, 81, 103, 180; personal freedom and, 161, 183; as primary prevention strategy, 39–42, 44, 47, 54, 157, 183–86; Protestant discourse and, 182; public health and, 2, 3, 4–5, 8, 9, 12; self-control and, 34–35, 39, 44, 53,

185; tradition and, 71–72; Ugandan interpretation, 80–81, 90–91, 95, 148–49; Ugandan personhood and, 6, 183; use of term, 11, 148–49. *See also* accountable subject; behavior change

individual choice, 100, 180

intentionality, 10, 126; abstinence and, 81–82, 93, 95, 96–97, 102; accountability and, 185; traditional morality and, 97–102; Ugandan interpretation of, 81–82, 95

interdependence: autonomy and, 14, 75–76; moral personhood and, 109–11; of spiritual/physical health, 112–17

International AIDS Conference (2000), 36

International AIDS Conference (2004), 35, 39–41

International Monetary Fund, 8

James, Erica, 32

Jezebel (biblical figure), 127

Kant, Immanuel, 14–15

Karlström, Mikael, 178, 266

Kato, David, 178

Keane, Webb, 89, 146–47, 211n30

kinship, 5–6, 57–58, 60, 74–76, 165, 169, 181

Klaits, Fred, 142–43

Kodesh, Neil, 12, 110

Kristeva, Julia, 175

kwabya lumbe (succession ceremonies), 113, 124–25

Laidlaw, James, 177

Lancet (journal), 37

landownership, 66, 199–200n18

lesbianism, 175–76

Li, Tania, 5

Livingston, Julie, 111, 115

Lord's Resistance Army (LRA), 167

love: faithful, 146–47; God's, 146; health and, 133–36; money and, 136–45; sincere, 146–48

LRA. *See* Lord's Resistance Army (LRA)

Lutz, Catherine, 134

Mair, Lucy, 66

marriage, 58–63; bridewealth exchange, 57–58, 60, 64–65, 70–71, 135, 142–43, 149–50, 164–65, 211n30; British common law and, 199n11; church, as status symbols, 212n34; customary law

marriage (cont.)
and, 199n11; faithfulness and, 130–33;
fortress imagery, 87–88; idealized love
and, 135; legal protections, 69–70;
monogamy, 61–63, 64–65, 72–73;
social change and, 63–66
Marriage and Divorce Bill, 69–70
Marshall, Ruth, 72
Martin, Emily, 109
Mauss, Marcel, 32
Mbembe, Achille, 174–75
Merry, Sally, 163
Miti, Jesumi, 65
monogamy, 61–63, 64–65, 72–73
moral authority, 4, 15–18, 23; cosmopolitan,
69–74; tradition and, 56–57
morality: African cultural values and, 72–73,
100; American evangelical models, 17;
behavior change and, 11–12; born-again
Christian, 3–4; collective, 65; crisis of,
63–66, 74; enacting, 181; overlapping
systems, 15; policy makers and, 7, 53;
politics of, 62; of power, 75; as proper
behavior, 89, 91; public health and,
4, 12–15, 133; rational choice and, 9;
sexual, 2, 3–4, 64, 71, 74, 82, 152, 157,
184, 208n24, 212n42; sexual rights and,
183–84; study of in ethnographies, 13;
traditional, criticism of, 100
Muehlebach, Andrea, 31
Museveni, Janet, 46–47, 48
Museveni, Yoweri, 10, 39–41, 42–43, 45, 47,
92, 178, 211n28
Mutebi. See Muwenda Mutebi II
Muwenda Mutebi II, 79, 92, 202n1
Mwanga, 165, 200n22, 213–14n11

naming, act of, 113–14
National Resistance Movement (NRM), 42
neoliberalism: accountability in, 5, 8, 10,
11, 12, 14, 16, 81, 103, 180; on behavior
change, 41, 44; defined, 8–9; freedom
and, 8–9, 103; human rights and,
176–79; personal empowerment in,
86–87, 103, 158, 176, 180
Nguyen, Vinh-Kim, 11, 36
night dancers. See basezi (night dancers)
nongovernmental organizations
(NGOs): access to services and, 6–7;
accountable subjects and, 157–58;
homosexual recruitment and, 172–73;
management of aid by, 10–11, 19, 33,
40, 47–49, 84

NRM. See National Resistance Movement
(NRM)
Nyerere, Julius, 42
Nyole ethnic group, 110

Obama, Barack, 157
occult, 15–16, 174–76, 205n20

Parikh, Shanti, 146
PEPFAR. See President's Emergency Plan
for AIDS Relief (PEPFAR)
personal accountability. See individual
accountability
personal empowerment: abstinence and,
86–87, 95–96, 105, 161; compassionate
conservatism on, 30; faithfulness
and, 153; moral worth of, 80; in
neoliberalism, 86–87, 103, 158, 176,
180; in public health policy, 2–3, 16,
24, 31; structural factors in, 183, 184;
Ugandan message of, 52–53, 181
personhood: African models of, 6–7, 12, 90,
162–63, 177, 182; health and, 109–11,
118; individual accountability and,
6, 183; moral, 5–6, 14, 81, 88, 90–92,
109–11, 125, 146–47, 163, 178; sexuality
and, 158–60, 159–60, 164–68, 179, 182;
in traditional culture, 90, 178
Peterson, Anne, 45–46
Peterson, Derek, 17, 59–60, 67
Petryna, Adriana, 11
Piot, Charles, 90
Piot, Peter, 35
polygamy, 62, 64
President's Emergency Plan for AIDS
Relief (PEPFAR): as abstinence and
faithfulness program, 9–10, 37, 79–80,
181, 184; compassion and accountability
in, 34–35; congressional debates over,
44–47; emphasis on faithfulness, 130,
151; funding, 3–4, 19, 35, 36–37, 44–47,
48–49, 157, 184; global response, 35–39;
introduction of, 27–30; on moral
behavior, 4–5, 35, 188n13, 194n37;
neoliberal policies and, 180; policy
guideline changes, 157; religious
activists and, 17; as self-help program,
2–3
privatization, 8, 10
public confession, 57, 66, 67–68
public health: ABC prevention plan, 37,
40, 44–45, 47, 48; accountability and,
3, 4–5, 8, 9, 12; behavior change

and, 45; discourses about love and,
133–36; healing practices in Africa,
12–13; morality and, 4, 12–15, 133;
use of term, 12. *See also* HIV/AIDS in
Uganda; President's Emergency Plan
for AIDS Relief (PEPFAR)

Reagan, Ronald, 27
Republican National Convention (1988), 31
respectability. *See ekitiibwa* (respectability)
revivalists. *See* East African Revival
Rose, Nikolas, 9
Rudnyckyj, Daromir, 9, 86–87
Ryan White Act (1990), 27

Samaritan's Purse, 49
secrecy, 174–76
self-control: abstinence and, 47, 79, 86,
88–89, 94–95, 100, 103, 116–17, 127, 130,
163–64; *ekitiibwa* (respectability) and,
91–92, 105; faith and, 86–87; individual
accountability and, 34–35, 39, 44, 53,
185; monogamy and, 64; moral agency
and, 6, 91; personal empowerment and,
181; public health programs on, 5, 8,
79; teaching, 197n72
self-empowerment. *See* personal
empowerment
sex education, 45, 49, 50
sexuality: accountability and, 80–81,
91, 181, 185–86; control of, 96, 103;
cultural context, 48; disciplined
subject, 88–89; freedom and, 165–68;
kinship roles and, 169–70; materiality
of, 152; in media, 94; models of, 93,
135; modern costs of, 93–97; in moral
personhood, 158–60, 159–60, 164–68,
179, 182; political/moral authority
over, 65, 68–69, 71, 75; predatory
male, 168; racist depictions, 135;
secretive, 174–76; self-restraint in,
91–92; sexual excess, 64; as social
advocacy topic, 158; spiritual/physical
costs of, 119–22; Western, history of,
89, 160; women's fashion and, 139. *See
also* homosexuality
sexual rights, 158–60, 170, 182–84
Shirati Jazz (band), 144
Simmel, Georg, 174
sincerity, 146–48
Smith, Shepherd, 45, 49
social activism, 17, 21–22, 57, 70–73, 157–58,
163. *See also* HIV/AIDS in Uganda

sodomy, 159
spiritual health, 111–17; deliverance prayer,
117–22, 123, 125–26, 127; relationships
and, 122–26; secrecy and, 173–76
Ssempa, Martin, 174
State of the Union address (G. W. Bush,
2003), 27–28, 30
Straight Talk Uganda, 43, 48, 50
succession ceremonies. *See kwabya lumbe*
(succession ceremonies)
sugar daddies/mommies, 131, 141, 152, 170
Summers, Carol, 68

taxation on foreign investment, 8
The AIDS Support Organisation (TASO),
43
Thomas, Lynn, 134
Thornton, Robert, 43, 44
Ticktin, Miriam, 11, 32, 36
Tobias, Randall, 37
traditional culture, 21; Christian politics
and, 57–58, 72; contested ideas of,
55–56; criticisms of, 97–102; faithfulness
in, 45–46; individual accountability,
71–72; missionaries on, 61–63; in
modern state, 55–58, 81; morality and
intentionality, 97–102; personhood in,
178; return to, 63–66

Uganda civil war, 55, 167
Uganda Youth Forum, 48
Ujamma reforms, 42
unemployment, 16, 86, 150–51
United Nations, 35–36, 37, 45
urbanization, 15, 56, 67, 93–97, 100, 172,
210n25
USAID, 28, 44, 45–46

Valentine's Day holiday, 106–7
volunteerism, 31–32, 34

Wardlow, Holly, 135
Weber, Max, 17
Wendland, Claire, 109
Whyte, Susan Reynolds, 110
witchcraft, 115, 176, 205n20
women's rights movement, 178, 195–96n53
World AIDS Day, 50, 130–31
World Bank, 8
World Health Organization, 1
World Vision, 28, 49

zero grazing, use of term, 43, 46